Problem Solving in Cardiology

Problem Solving in
Cardiology

H. S. LIM
Haemostasis Thrombosis and Vascular Biology Unit, University Department of Medicine,
City Hospital, Birmingham, UK

G. Y. H. LIP
Haemostasis Thrombosis and Vascular Biology Unit, University Department of Medicine,
City Hospital, Birmingham, UK

CLINICAL PUBLISHING

OXFORD

CLINICAL PUBLISHING
an imprint of Atlas Medical Publishing Ltd
Oxford Centre for Innovation
Mill Street, Oxford OX2 0JX, UK

tel: +44 1865 811116
fax: +44 1865 251550

e mail: info@clinicalpublishing.co.uk
web: www.clinicalpublishing.co.uk

Distributed in USA and Canada by:
Clinical Publishing
30 Amberwood Parkway
Ashland OH 44805 USA
tel: 800-247-6553 (toll free within US and Canada)
fax: 419-281-6883
email: order@bookmasters.com

Distributed in UK and Rest of World by:
Marston Book Services Ltd
PO Box 269
Abingdon
Oxon OX14 4YN
UK
tel: +44 1235 465500
fax: +44 1235 465555
email: trade.orders@marston.co.uk

© Atlas Medical Publishing Ltd 2010

First published 2010

All rights reserved. No part of this publication may be reproduced, stored in a retrieval system, or transmitted, in any form or by any means, without the prior permission in writing of Clinical Publishing or Atlas Medical Publishing Ltd.

Although every effort has been made to ensure that all owners of copyright material have been acknowledged in this publication, we would be glad to acknowledge in subsequent reprints or editions any omissions brought to our attention.

Clinical Publishing and Atlas Medical Publishing Ltd bear no responsibility for the persistence or accuracy of URLs for external or third-party internet websites referred to in this publication, and do not guarantee that any content on such websites is, or will remain, accurate or appropriate.

A catalogue record for this book is available from the British Library.

ISBN 13   978 1 84692 046 2
ISBN e-book   978 1 84692 618 1

The publisher makes no representation, express or implied, that the dosages in this book are correct. Readers must therefore always check the product information and clinical procedures with the most up-to-date published product information and data sheets provided by the manufacturers and the most recent codes of conduct and safety regulations. The authors and the publisher do not accept any liability for any errors in the text or for the misuse or misapplication of material in this work.

Project manager: Gavin Smith, GPS Publishing Solutions, Herts, UK
Typeset by Phoenix Photosetting, Chatham, UK
Printed by Marston Book Services, Abingdon, Oxon, UK

Contents

Abbreviations   vii

SECTION 1   Primary Prevention

1. Risk stratification and guidelines   1
2. Antihypertensive therapy   7
3. Dyslipidaemia   12

SECTION 2   Coronary Artery Disease

4. Assessment of stable angina   17
5. Treatment of stable angina   24
6. Management of acute coronary syndrome   29
7. Initial management of ST elevation myocardial infarction   36
8. Hypotension in acute myocardial infarction   44
9. Cardiogenic shock   48
10. Peri-infarct arrhythmia   54
11. Secondary prevention (lifestyle, risk factors and drug treatment)   59

SECTION 3   Arterial Disease and Syncope

12. Aortic dissection   65
13. Hypertensive emergencies   70
14. Neurocardiogenic syncope   74
15. Cardiac tumours   79

SECTION 4   Valvular Heart Disease

16. Mitral stenosis   83
17. Mitral regurgitation   87
18. Aortic stenosis   92
19. Aortic regurgitation   97
20. Infective endocarditis   100

SECTION 5 Cardiac Arrhythmias

21. Narrow complex tachycardia   107
22. Atrial fibrillation   113
23. Broad complex tachycardia   120
24. Bradyarrhythmia   126
25. Sudden cardiac death   131

SECTION 6 Cardiomyopathy and Pericardial Disease

26. Hypertrophic cardiomyopathy   137
27. Dilated cardiomyopathy   142
28. Restrictive cardiomyopathy   147
29. Pericarditis   153
30. Pericardial effusion   157

SECTION 7 Congenital Heart Disease

31. Ventricular septal defect   161
32. Atrial septal defect and patent foramen ovale   165
33. Tetralogy of Fallot   170
34. Coarctation of aorta   174
35. Contraception in congenital heart disease   177

SECTION 8 Pregnancy and Heart Disease

36. Valve disease and pregnancy   183
37. Prosthetic valve and anticoagulation   186
38. Hypertension in pregnancy   189

SECTION 9 Cardiac Disease and Operative Risk

39. Perioperative risk stratification and β-blocker   195

General index   201

Abbreviations

4S	Scandinavian Simvastatin Survival Study	CaCC	calcium-activated chloride channel
ACCORD	Action to Control Cardiovascular Risk in Diabetes	CAPRIE	Clopidogrel versus Aspirin in Patients at Risk of Ischaemic Events
ACE	angiotensin-converting enzyme	CAST	Cardiac Arrhythmia Suppression Trial
ADVANCE	Action in Diabetes and Vascular Disease: Preterax and Diamicron Modified Release Controlled Evaluation	CCS	Canadian Cardiovascular Society
		CF	cystic fibrosis
		CHADS	Congestive heart failure, Hypertension, Age over 75, Diabetes, Stroke/TIA
AF	atrial fibrillation		
ALLHAT	Antihypertensive and Lipid-Lowering Treatment to Prevent Heart Attack Trial	CK	creatine kinase
		CO	cardiac output
		COMMIT	Clopidogrel and Metoprolol in Myocardial Infarction Trial
ARBITER 6-HALTS	Arterial Biology for the Investigation of the Treatment Effects of Reducing Cholesterol 6: HDL and LDL Treatment Strategies in Atherosclerosis	COPE	Colchicine for Acute Pericarditis
		CORE	Colchicine for Recurrent Pericarditis
		COURAGE	Clinical Outcomes Utilizing Revascularization and Aggressive Drug Evaluation
ASCOT-LLA	Anglo-Scandinavian Cardiac Outcomes Trial – Lipid Lowering Arm		
		CT	computed tomography
ASD	atrial septal defect	CURE	Clopidogrel in Unstable Angina to Prevent Recurrent Events
ATHENA	A Placebo-Controlled, Double Blind, Parallel Arm Trial to Assess the Efficacy of Dronedarone 400 mg bid for the Prevention of Cardiovascular Hospitalization or Death from Any Cause in Patients with Atrial Fibrillation/Atrial Flutter	CURE	Clopidogrel in Unstable Angina to Prevent Recurrent Events
		CVD	cardiovascular disease
		CVP	central venous pressure
		DANAMI-2	Danish Trial in Acute Myocardial Infarction-2
		DIGAMI	Diabetes Mellitus Insulin-Glucose Infusion in Acute Myocardial Infarction
AV	atrioventricular		
AVNRT	atrioventricular nodal re-entry tachycardia	DINAMIT	Defibrillator in Acute Myocardial Infarction Trial
AVR	aortic valve replacement	ECG	electrocardiogram
AVRT	atrioventricular re-entry tachycardia	EF	ejection fraction
		EGSYS	Evaluation of Guidelines in Syncope Study
A-VSaO$_2$	difference between arterial and mixed venous oxygen saturations		
		ENaC	epithelial sodium channel
BD	twice daily	EPHESUS	Eplerenone Post-Acute Myocardial Infarction Heart Failure Efficacy and Survival Study
BMI	body mass index		
BP	blood pressure		
CABG	coronary artery bypass graft		

ESD	end-systolic dimension
EUROPA	EUropean trial on Reduction Of cardiac events with Perindopril in stable coronary Artery disease
FINESSE	Facilitated Intervention with Enhanced Reperfusion Speed to Stop Events
FRISC	Fragmin during Instability in Coronary Artery Disease
GISSI	Gruppo Italiano per lo Studio della Sopravvivenza nell'Infarto Miocardico
GRACE	Global Registry of Acute Coronary Events
GTN	glyceryl trinitrate
HACEK	Haemophilus, Actinobacillus, Cardiobacterium, Eikenella, Kingella
HCM	hypertrophic cardiomopathy
HDL	high-density lipoprotein
HDU	high dependency unit
HMG-CoA	3-hydroxy-3-methylglutaryl-coenzyme A
HOPE	Heart Outcomes Prevention Evaluation
HR	hazard ratio
HYVET	Hypertension in the Very Elderly Trial
IABP	intra-aortic balloon pump
ICD	implantable cardioverter defibrillator
Ig	immunoglobulin
INSTEAD	INvestigation of STEnt Grafts in Patients with Type B Aortic Dissection
IONA	Impact of Nicorandil in Angina
ISIS-2	Second International Study of Infarct Survival
ISSUE 2	International Study on Syncope of Uncertain Etiology 2
IVC	inferior vena cava
JBS	Joint British Societies
JUPITER	Justification for the Use of Statins in Prevention: an Intervention Trial Evaluating Rosuvastatin
LADIP	Loire-Ardèche-Drôme-Isère-Puy-de-Dôme
LBBB	left bundle branch block
LDL	low-density lipoprotein
LMW	low molecular weight
LV	left ventricular
LVEDD	left ventricular end-diastolic diameter
LVEDP	left ventricular end-diastolic pressure
LVEF	left ventricular ejection fraction
LVESD	left ventricular end-systolic diameter
LVH	left ventricular hypertension
LVOT	left ventricular outflow tract
MADIT	Multicenter Automatic Defibrillator Implantation Trial
MBL	mannose binding lectin
MERLIN TIMI-36	Metabolic Efficiency with Ranolazine for Less Ischemia in Non-ST Elevation Acute Coronary Syndromes
MI	myocardial infarction
MIST	Migraine Intervention with STARFlex Technology
MR	mitral regurgitation
MRI	magnetic resonance imaging
MRSA	methicillin-resistant *Staphylococcus aureus*
NICE	National Institute for Clinical Excellence
NO	nitric oxide
NSAID	non-steroidal anti-inflammatory drug
NSTEMI	non-ST elevation myocardial infarction
NSVT	non-sustained ventricular tachycardia
NYHA	New York Heart Association
OD	once daily
PACE	Promoting Healthy Ageing with Cognitive Exercise
PCI	percutaneous coronary intervention
PCO_2	partial pressure of carbon dioxide
PCWP	pulmonary capillary wedge pressure
PDA	patent ductus arteriosus
PEA	pulseless electrical activity
PEFR	peak expiratory flow rate
PFO	patent foramen ovale
POISE	Perioperative Ischaemia Evaluation trial
POST	Prevention of Syncope Trial
PPCI	primary percutaneous coronary intervention
PTCA	percutaneous transluminal coronary angioplasty
RA	right atrium

RALES	Randomized Aldosterone Evaluation Study	SVC	superior vena cava
RCRI	Revised Cardiac Risk Index	SVR	systemic vascular resistance
REACT	Rescue Angioplasty Versus Conservative Treatment or Repeat Thrombolysis	SYNPACE	SYNcope and PACing trial
		TC	total cholesterol
		TIMI	Thrombolysis in Myocardial Infarction
RV	right ventricular	t-PA	tissue plasminogen activator
RVEDP	right ventricular end-diastolic pressure	TRITON TIMI-38	TRial to assess Improvement in Therapeutic Outcomes by optimising platelet iNhibition with prasugrel – Thrombolysis In Myocardial Infarction 38
RVSP	right ventricular systolic pressure		
SAVE PACE	Search AV Extension and Managed Ventricular Pacing for Promoting Atrioventricular Conduction		
		UFH	unfractionated heparin
SAM	systolic anterior motion	UKPDS	United Kingdom Prospective Diabetes Study
SBP	systolic blood pressure		
SCD-HeFT	Sudden Cardiac Death in Heart Failure Trial	VPS	Vasovagal Pacemaker Study
		VSD	ventricular septal defect
SHOCK	Should we emergently revascularize Occuded Coronaries for shocK	VT	ventricular tachycardia
		WHO	World Health Organization
SR	slow release	WOSCOPS	West of Scotland Coronary Prevention Study
STEMI	ST elevation myocardial infarction		

SECTION ONE 01

Primary Prevention

1   Risk stratification and guidelines
2   Antihypertensive therapy
3   Dyslipidaemia

PROBLEM

1 Risk stratification and guidelines

Case History

A 65-year-old man attended a routine clinic assessment following his recent retirement and was found to have a serum total cholesterol of 6.1 mmol/l. His fasting triglyceride was measured at 1.6 mmol/l, high-density lipoprotein cholesterol at 1.0 mmol/l (total : high-density lipoprotein cholesterol ratio >6) and fasting plasma glucose was normal. His blood pressure was measured at 150/84 mmHg in the clinic. He has a waist circumference of 94 cm. He has no past medical history and does not take any regular medications. He does not smoke cigarettes. He insisted that he adheres rigorously to a healthy diet with five portions of fruits and vegetables daily, and since his retirement, has also been cycling and playing golf at least three times per week.

What are the indications and targets for lipid-lowering therapy?

Does he need treatment for his blood pressure?

Background

This man does not have documented cardiovascular disease (CVD). Therefore, treatment will be aimed at primary prevention of cardiovascular events. Lipid-lowering therapy with statins (HMG-CoA reductase inhibitors) has been shown to reduce cardiovascular events in the setting of primary prevention in the WOSCOPS (West of Scotland Coronary Prevention Study) and ASCOT-LLA (Anglo-Scandinavian Cardiac Outcomes Trial – Lipid Lowering Arm) studies. The latter randomized patients with hypertension without overt coronary heart disease and total cholesterol of <6.5 mmol/l to atorvastatin

10 mg or placebo, and was terminated early because of significant reductions in cardiovascular events compared with placebo (Figure 1.1).

The recent Joint British Societies (JBS) guidelines recommend therapeutic intervention in the context of primary prevention in patients with:

- diabetes mellitus;
- blood pressure >160/100 mmHg or lesser degree of hypertension with evidence of target organ damage;
- total cholesterol : high-density lipoprotein cholesterol ratio >6;
- familial hypercholesterolaemia, or;
- an estimated CVD risk of >20% over 10 years.

Therefore, the measurement of lipid levels should be performed as part of an overall cardiovascular risk assessment. Monitoring of lipid levels remains relevant, as the benefit of statin therapy is proportional to the reduction in cholesterol, in particular low-density lipoprotein cholesterol. Total cholesterol of <4 mmol/l or low-density lipoprotein cholesterol of <2 mmol/l are the recommended targets. Fasting lipid measurements are generally not required for total cholesterol measurements, although serum triglycerides may be affected by dietary intake.

The second JBS guidelines now recommend a move towards the more global CVD risk, which includes the risk of stroke (fatal/non-fatal stroke, intracerebral haemorrhage and transient ischaemic attack) in addition to coronary events. The new CVD charts are based on the Framingham risk function and specify three levels of 10-year CVD risk: ≥30%, ≥20% and ≤10%, which are represented by three colour bands on the chart (Figure 1.2). Lipid-lowering therapy (statin) is recommended in this case, as his 10-year cardiovascular risk is >20% based on the charts.

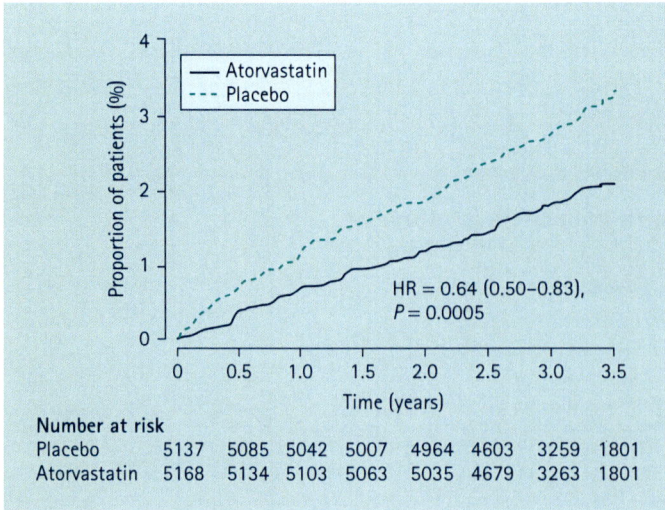

Figure 1.1 Cumulative incidence of fatal and non-fatal coronary events from the ASCOT-LLA study (Anglo-Scandinavian Cardiac Outcomes Trial - Lipid Lowering Arm). HR, hazard ratio.

01 Risk stratification and guidelines

Does he need treatment for his blood pressure?

The need for antihypertensive treatment is similarly guided by more than just absolute blood pressure measurements. In this man's case, blood pressure should be rechecked to confirm persistently elevated blood pressure. In addition to the assessment of cardiovascular risk (as discussed previously), evidence of target organ damage (e.g. retinopathy, proteinuria, evidence of left ventricular hypertrophy) should also be sought. The presence of target organ damage implies an elevated cardiovascular risk and the need for intervention.

The targeting of antihypertensive treatment at absolute (CVD) risk is underpinned by evidence from meta-analyses of outcome trials. These studies show that the relative risk

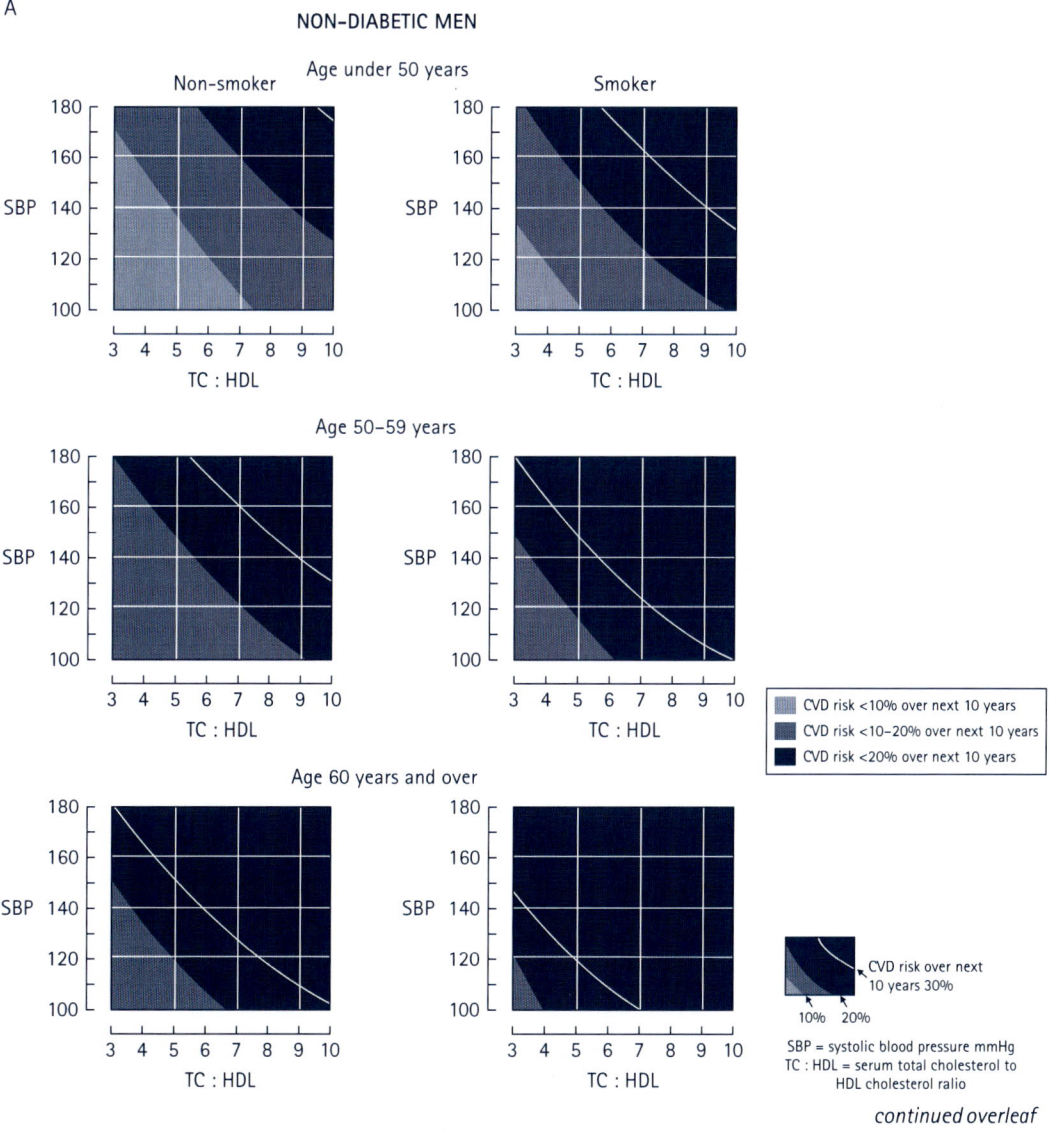

continued overleaf

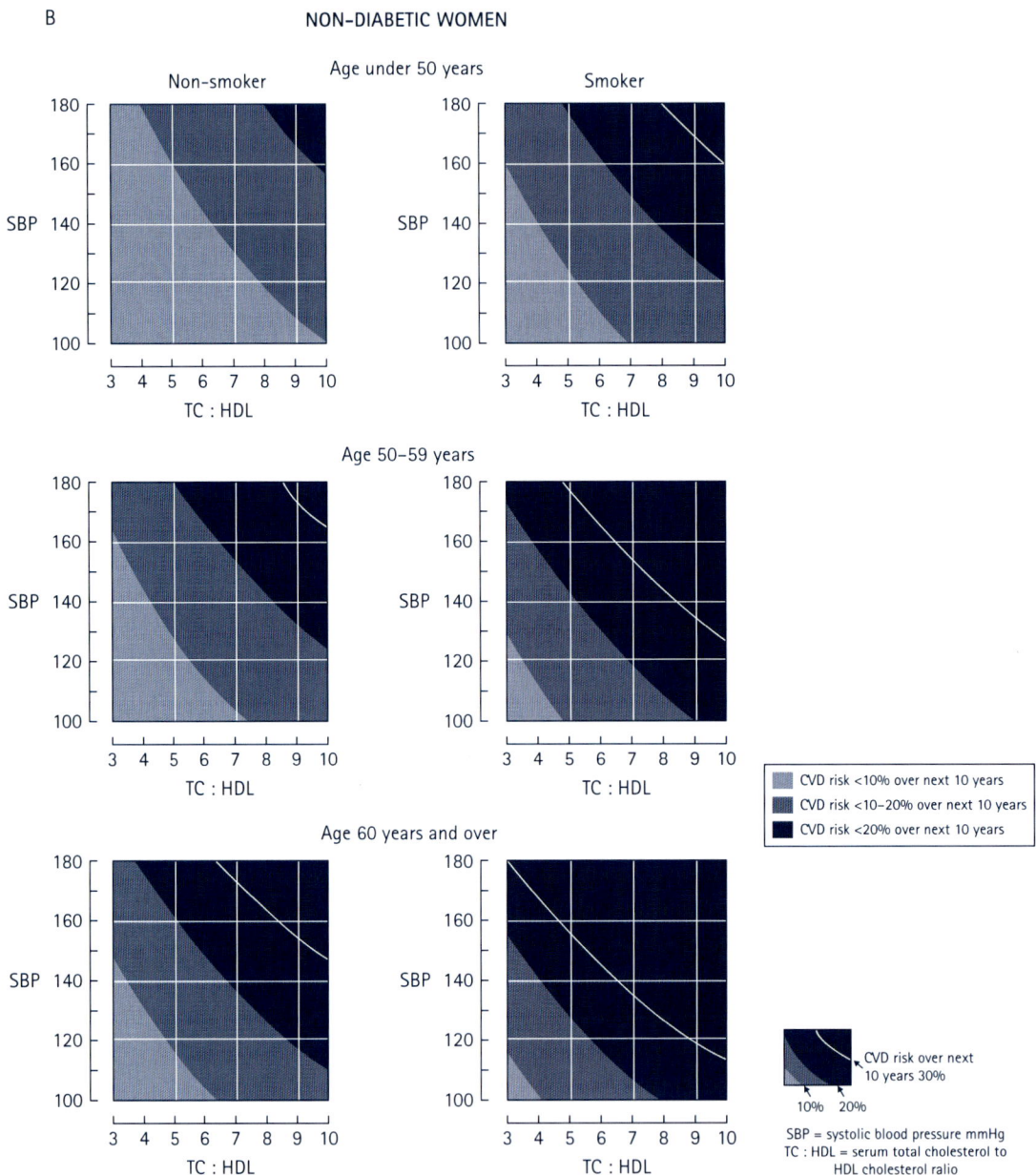

Figure 1.2 Smokers and non-smokers. (A) Non-diabetic men; (B) non-diabetic women. CVD, cardiovascular disease; HDL, high-density lipoprotein; SBP, systolic blood pressure; TC, total cholesterol.

reduction by antihypertensive treatment is approximately constant, with a 38% reduction in stroke and 16% reduction in coronary events. Even in patients with mild hypertension, treatment reduces cardiovascular complications by approximately 25%, but as the absolute risk is low, the absolute benefit will be low, which translates into a higher number needed to treat and greater costs to prevent one cardiovascular event. In contrast, treatment of patients at a 10-year CVD risk of ≥20% results in greater absolute benefit, which corresponds to a lower number needed to treat for 5 years of 40 – this means treatment of 40 patients for 5 years to prevent one cardiovascular complication. Hence, decisions on treatment at lower levels of CVD risk will be influenced by the patient's attitude to treatment and the benefit anticipated from treatment.

Current practice guidelines recommend that all patients with average BP 140–159 or 90–99 mmHg should be offered antihypertensive drug treatment if (Figure 1.3):

- there is any complication of hypertension or target organ damage, or diabetes;
- the 10-year CVD risk is ≥20% despite advice on non-pharmacological measures.

Antihypertensive therapy is recommended if hypertension is confirmed by repeat blood pressure measurement.

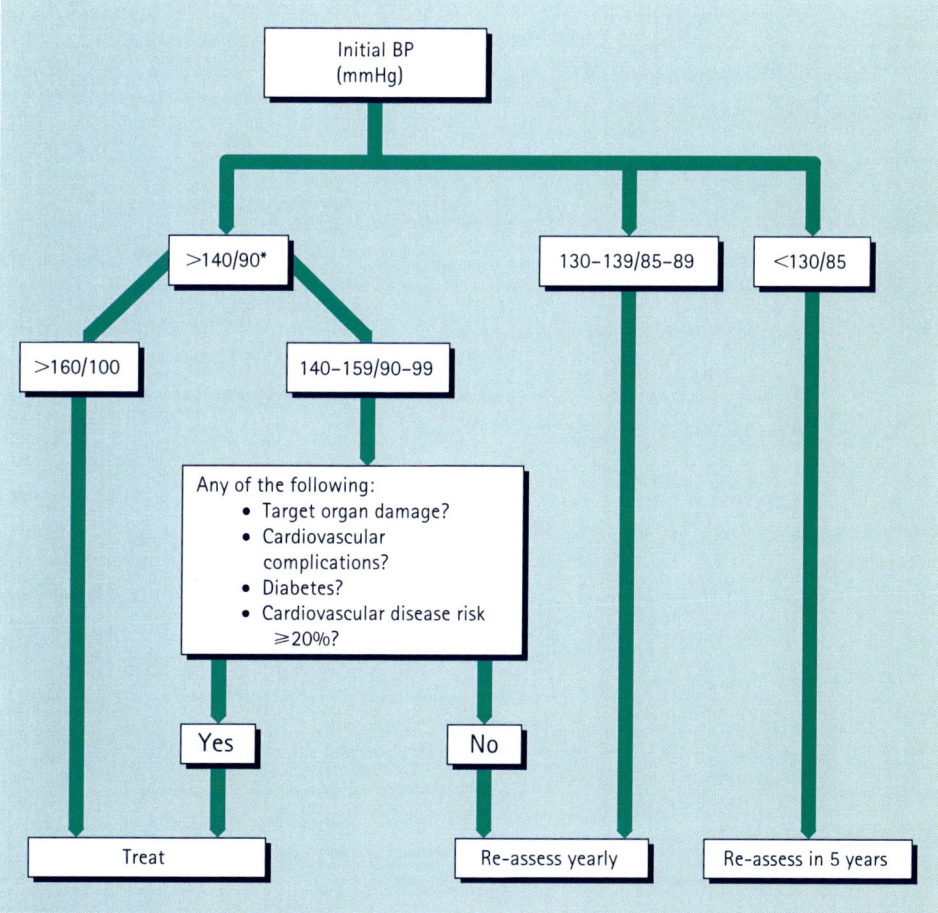

Figure 1.3 Blood pressure (BP) threshold for intervention. *If initial BP >180/110, confirm over 1–2 weeks unless malignant phase hypertension (if initial BP 160–179/100–109, confirm over 3–4 weeks then treat; if initial BP 140–159/90–99, confirm over 12 weeks then treat).

Recent Developments

The assessment and treatment of cardiovascular risk has evolved from one targeting individual risk factors to a global multifactorial approach. This is clearly supported by the benefit of lipid-lowering therapy in patients with hypertension (ASCOT-LLA) and diabetes mellitus (Collaborative Atorvastatin Diabetes Study). In contrast to glycaemic reduction in diabetes, which yielded only a modest reduction in cardiovascular events, a global multifactorial intervention strategy has been shown to significantly reduce cardiovascular morbidity and mortality.

Conclusion

Cardiovascular risk increases with increasing blood pressure level, and in association with other risk factors such as diabetes mellitus and hypercholesterolaemia. This is the basis for using a multiple risk factor approach to cardiovascular risk assessment (Figure 1.2). Indeed, the threshold for treatment of high blood pressure is based not on absolute blood pressure measurement alone, but in conjunction with other risk factors and cardiovascular risk (Figure 1.3).

Further Reading

JBS 2: Joint British Societies' guidelines on prevention of cardiovascular disease in clinical practice. *Heart* 2005; **91**: 1–52.

Sever PS, Dahlof B, Poulter NR, *et al.* Prevention of coronary and stroke events with atorvastatin in hypertensive patients who have average or lower-than-average cholesterol concentrations, in the Anglo-Scandinavian Cardiac Outcomes Trial – Lipid Lowering Arm (ASCOT-LLA): a multicentre randomized controlled trial. *Lancet* 2003; **361**: 1149–58.

Williams B, Poulter NR, Brown MJ, *et al.* Guidelines for management of hypertension: report of the fourth working party of the British Hypertension Society. *J Hum Hypertens* 2004; **18**: 139–85.

02 Antihypertensive therapy

PROBLEM

Case History

A 76-year-old man has two blood pressure measurements taken 8 weeks apart, which confirm a persistently elevated blood pressure of 166/94 mmHg. He is aware of the need for blood pressure-lowering treatment in view of his hypertension and cardiovascular risk. He has impaired fasting glycaemia but no history of cardiovascular disease.

How is hypertension graded?

Which antihypertensive agent should he be treated with?

Background

How is hypertension graded?

The grading of hypertension has evolved over time as data on the association between blood pressure and cardiovascular events accumulated. The current grading of hypertension includes a category of 'high-normal' and is outlined in Table 2.1.

Which antihypertensive agent should he be treated with?

The choice of first-line antihypertensive therapy has been the subject of a number of clinical studies. The ALLHAT (Antihypertensive and Lipid-Lowering Treatment to Prevent Heart Attack Trial) study of >40 000 patients is the largest study to date and compared a thiazide diuretic (chlorthalidone), a calcium channel blocker (amlodipine), an angiotensin-converting enzyme (ACE) inhibitor (lisinopril) and an α-blocker (doxazosin) as a first-line agent in the treatment of hypertension. The doxazosin arm was terminated earlier due to an excess of a combined endpoint of cardiovascular events

Table 2.1 Blood pressure classification

Blood pressure category	Systolic blood pressure (mmHg)	Diastolic blood pressure (mmHg)
Normal	<120	<80
High–normal	135–139	85–89
Mild (grade 1)	140–159	90–99
Moderate (grade 2)	160–179	100–110
Severe (grade 3)	>180	>110

(particularly heart failure and stroke) compared with chlorthalidone, which was confirmed in a subsequent analysis. There was no difference in the primary outcome of fatal and non-fatal myocardial infarction and all-cause mortality in the lisinopril and amlodipine arms compared with chlorthalidone. Hence, thiazide diuretic, ACE inhibitor and calcium channel blockers are acceptable first-line antihypertensive agents. The choice of antihypertensive agent for individual patients should take into account the presence and absence of compelling indications and contraindications (Table 2.2).

In contrast, recent data have challenged the efficacy of the β-blocker atenolol compared with the other classes of antihypertensive therapy. The ASCOT (Anglo-Scandinavian Cardiac Outcomes Trial) study with 19 257 patients followed-up for a median of 5.5 years demonstrated significantly fewer cardiovascular events and lower all-cause mortality among patients randomized to the amlodipine–perindopril compared with the atenolol–bendroflumethiazide based treatment. These data led to a review by the Guideline Development Group at the National Institute of Clinical Excellence, which concluded that β-blockers should not be used as first-line treatment for hypertension in the absence of compelling indications (Figure 2.1).

However, β-blockers may still be considered in younger patients intolerant of ACE inhibitors or angiotensin II antagonists, of child-bearing potential (potentially teratogenic effects) and patients with high sympathetic drive. If β-blockers are used in these

Table 2.2 Compelling indications and contraindications

Class of drugs	Compelling indications	Contraindications
α-blockers	Benign prostatic hyperplasia	Urinary incontinence
Angiotensin-converting enzyme inhibitors	Heart failure, left ventricular dysfunction or established coronary heart disease, type 1 diabetic nephropathy, secondary stroke prevention (with thiazide)	Pregnancy, renovascular disease
Angiotensin receptor blocker	Angiotensin-converting enzyme inhibitor intolerance (heart failure), type 2 diabetic nephropathy, hypertension with left ventricular hypertrophy	Pregnancy, renovascular disease
β-blockers	Myocardial infarction, angina, heart failure	Asthma or chronic obstructive pulmonary disease, heart block
Dihydropyridine calcium channel blockers	Elderly patients, isolated systolic hypertension	–
Rate-limiting (non-dihydropyridine) calcium channel blockers	Angina	Heart block, heart failure
Thiazide diuretics	Elderly patients, isolated systolic hypertension, heart failure, secondary stroke prevention	Gout

Angiotensin-converting enzyme inhibitors and angiotensin II antagonists should be used with caution in patients with renal impairment; angiotensin-converting enzyme inhibitors and angiotensin II antagonists may be preferred in patients at high risk of developing diabetes (e.g. glucose intolerance, metabolic syndrome and family history of diabetes).
The use of β-blockers in heart failure may lead to transient deterioration in symptoms.
Thiazides may precipitate gout and concomitant allopurinol should be considered.

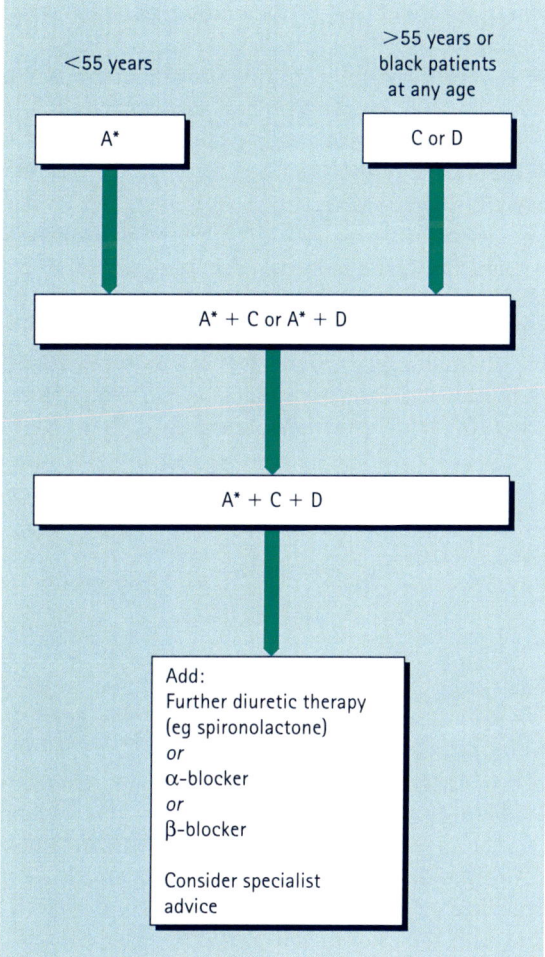

Figure 2.1 Algorithm for the treatment of hypertension (NICE update 2006). A, angiotensin-converting enzyme (ACE) inhibitors (*or angiotensin antagonist if ACE inhibitor intolerant); C, calcium channel blocker; D, thiazide diuretic. β-blockers are not preferred initial therapy for hypertension but are an alternative to A in patients <55 years in whom A is not tolerated or is contraindicated (includes women of child-bearing potential). Black patients are only those of African or Caribbean descent. In the absence of evidence, all other patients should be treated as non-black.

patients, a calcium channel blocker (not thiazide) should be added if additional antihypertensive treatment is needed to avoid the increased risk of diabetes with β-blocker–thiazide diuretic combination. The risk of diabetes may be particularly relevant in patients of South Asian origin and patients with impaired glucose tolerance or impaired fasting glycaemia, who are already at increased risk of developing diabetes.

In this case, a dihydropyridine calcium channel blocker, such as amlodipine, would be reasonable in view of his age, systolic hypertension and impaired fasting glycaemia. Blood pressure should be treated to a target of 140/85 mmHg. An ACE inhibitor or angiotensin receptor blocker may be added for further blood pressure control if the target is not achieved.

The majority of patients with hypertension will require more than one antihypertensive agent. Some experts have recommended the use of combination therapy as first-line agents in patients with systolic blood pressure of over 160 mmHg since monotherapy, regardless of the agent used, is unlikely to reduce the systolic blood pressure to the treatment target. Indeed, combination tablets may improve compliance with treatment and should certainly be considered when patients are established on two or more antihypertensive agents. Currently available combination tablets include thiazide–ACE inhibitor combinations and calcium channel blocker–angiotensin receptor blocker combinations.

Importantly, antihypertensive therapy should not be withheld because of advanced age. Although there was initial concern with blood pressure lowering in the elderly, these concerns are largely dispelled by the recent HYVET (Hypertension in the Very Elderly Trial) study. The HYVET study included 3845 patients with hypertension over the age of 80 years and was terminated early due to significant reductions in strokes and all-cause mortality with blood pressure reduction (using a combination of indapamide and perindopril).

Recent Developments

Aliskiren, the first in the class of drugs dubbed direct renin inhibitors has recently been approved for the treatment of hypertension. The effect of this new antihypertensive agent on morbidity and mortality has yet to be tested in large randomized trials, but a number of clinical studies have confirmed the efficacy of aliskiren in reducing blood pressure and albuminuria. The blood pressure-lowering effects appear to be comparable with other antihypertensive agents (e.g. ACE inhibitors and calcium channel blockers) and may even be superior to thiazide diuretics. The blood pressure-lowering effects appear to be synergistic with calcium channel blockers and thiazide diuretics. Aliskiren also appears to be well tolerated with the rates of side effects comparable with placebo. Hence, aliskiren may be considered in patients with uncontrolled hypertension on conventional therapy.

The recent Action in Diabetes and Vascular Disease: Preterax and Diamicron MR Controlled Evaluation (ADVANCE) study compared fixed dose perindopril-indapamide versus placebo in patients with type-2 diabetes. The treatment arm achieved a systolic blood pressure of about 135 mmHg compared to 140 mmHg in the placebo group. Total mortality was lower in the perindopril-indapamide group compared to placebo (7.3% vs 8.5%) over 4.3 years, with fewer coronary events, reduced progression of nephropathy and microalbuminuria.

This was followed by the Action to Control Cardiovascular Risk in Diabetes (ACCORD) trial compared intensive blood pressure lowering to a target of less than 120 mmHg (systolic) versus conventional target of 140 mmHg in 4733 patients with type-2 diabetes. Although there was a small absolute reduction in stroke (0.32% vs 0.53%), there were significantly more adverse events related to intensive blood pressure reduction (3.3% vs 1.3%, $P < 0.001$). There was no difference in total mortality. These data suggest that there may be little benefit in lowering systolic blood pressure below 135 mmHg in patients with diabetes.

Conclusion

The pharmacological treatment of hypertension has evolved considerably over the years. Recent randomized trials have compared old drugs against the newer ones. The current treatment algorithm reflects the results of these studies. In uncomplicated hypertension, ACE inhibitors (or angiotensin receptor blockers), thiazide diuretics or calcium channel blockers are recommended first-line agents. Their use in combination offers further blood pressure reduction. The presence of compelling indications or contraindications should also be considered in selecting the appropriate antihypertensive treatment.

Further Reading

ACCORD Study Group. Effects of intensive blood pressure control in type-2 diabetes mellitus. *N Engl J Med* 2010; **362**: 1575–85.

Dahlof B, Sever P, Poulter NR, *et al.* Prevention of cardiovascular events with an antihypertensive regimen of amlodipine adding perindopril as required versus atenolol adding bendroflumethiazide as required, in the Anglo-Scandinavian Cardiac Outcomes Trial-Blood Pressure Lowering Arm (ASCOT-BPLA): a multicentre randomized controlled trial. *Lancet* 2005; **366**: 895–906.

Lindholm LH, Carlberg B, Samuelsson O. Should beta blockers remain first choice in the treatment of primary hypertension? A meta-analysis. *Lancet* 2005; **366**: 1545–53.

National Collaborating Centre for Chronic Conditions. *Hypertension: management of hypertension in adults in primary care: partial update.* London: Royal College of Physicians, 2006.

Patel A, MacMahon S, Chalmers J, Neal B, Woodward M, et al. Effects of a fixed combination of perindopril and indapamide on macrovascular and microvascular outcomes in patiets with type-2 diabetes mellitus (the ADVANCE trial). *Lancet* 2007; **370**: 829–40.

The ALLHAT Officers and Coordinators for the ALLHAT Collaborative Research Group. Major outcomes in high-risk hypertensive patients randomized to angiotensin-converting enzyme inhibitor or calcium channel blocker vs diuretic: The Anti-hypertensive and Lipid Lowering Treatment to Prevent Heart Attack Trial (ALLHAT). *JAMA* 2002; **288**: 2981–97.

Williams B, Poulter NR, Brown MJ, *et al.* Guidelines for management of hypertension: report of the fourth working party of the British Hypertension Society. *J Hum Hypertens* 2004; **18**: 139–85.

PROBLEM

03 Dyslipidaemia

Case History

A 54-year-old South Asian man with hypertension and a 2-year history of type 2 diabetes mellitus attended a routine clinical assessment. He had a waist circumference of 90 cm. He did not have documented cardiovascular disease. His total cholesterol was 4.6 mmol/l, fasting triglyceride 4.8 mmol/l, high-density lipoprotein (HDL) cholesterol 0.8 mmol/l and HbA1c 7.9%. He is currently on simvastatin 40 mg daily in addition to his antihypertensive and oral hypoglycaemic agents.

Is this man's lipid profile satisfactory?

What are the current recommendations for the treatment of dyslipidaemia?

Background

This man has multiple cardiovascular risk factors and fulfils the International Diabetes Federation criteria for the metabolic syndrome (Table 3.1). This clinical syndrome describes the frequent coalition of multiple risk factors and identifies individuals at high risk of cardiovascular events. However, the definition of metabolic syndrome, particu-

Table 3.1 International Diabetes Federation definition of metabolic syndrome
Central obesity
Waist circumference – ethnicity specific
Plus any two of: • Raised triglycerides (>1.7 mmol/l)* • Reduced high-density lipoprotein cholesterol (<1.03 mmol/l for men, <1.3 mmol/l for women)* • Raised blood pressure (systolic ≥130 mmHg, diastolic ≥85 mmHg or diagnosed hypertension) • Raised fasting plasma glucose (≥5.6 mmol/l or diagnosed type 2 diabetes)
Ethnic group and waist circumference
Europids (men >94 cm; women >80 cm)
Chinese and South Asians (men >90 cm; women >80 cm)
Japanese (men >85 cm; women >90 cm)
Ethnic south and central Americans (use South Asian recommendations)
Sub-Saharan Africans (use European data)
Eastern Mediterranean and Middle-East population (use European data)

larly in different ethnic groups, the clinical value and incorporation of metabolic syndrome into clinical practice have been the subject of considerable debate. Current guidelines do not recommend the use of metabolic syndrome over conventional risk estimation (based on Framingham risk scoring) for the assessment of cardiovascular risk.

Based on conventional risk assessment, this man's estimated cardiovascular risk is well in excess of 20% over 10 years. Statin therapy has been shown to reduce the risk of major vascular events (fatal/non-fatal myocardial infarction and stroke) by 21%, which in this case, would leave significant residual cardiovascular risk. Treatment of his dyslipidaemia may reduce this risk further. Of note, epidemiological studies suggest that South Asians in the UK have about 40% excess risk of coronary disease, but the treatment targets have not been modified to take this into consideration. Hence, this man requires further treatment for his dyslipidaemia.

What are the current recommendations for the treatment of dyslipidaemia?

Lifestyle modification with dietary intervention, increasing physical activity and weight loss should be offered to all patients at high cardiovascular risk. However, lifestyle intervention should be complemented by pharmacological treatment in high-risk patients. Statin therapy, with the primary aim of lowering total and low-density lipoprotein (LDL) cholesterol is the first-line lipid-lowering treatment. Simvastatin 40 mg OD has been recommended as first-line treatment by recent National Institute for Clinical Excellence (NICE) guidance, but in the absence of diabetes or metabolic syndrome, no specific treatment targets were set for primary prevention of cardiovascular events. Indeed, further lipid testing was not routinely recommended by NICE guidance in these patients with uncomplicated hypercholesterolaemia in the setting of primary prevention. An alternative statin, such as pravastatin (less metabolism via the cytochrome P450 pathway) or lower dose statin, may be used if simvastatin 40 mg is not tolerated.

However, the need for more intensive lipid management has been recognized in patients with diabetes and metabolic syndrome. Although a statin remains the first-line treatment, unlike recommendations for people with 'uncomplicated' hyperlipidaemia (e.g. without vascular disease, diabetes, albuminuria or metabolic syndrome), the total and LDL cholesterol should be treated to a target of 4 mmol/l and 2 mmol/l respectively. The doses and associated reduction in LDL cholesterol are listed in Table 3.2. An increase in the dose of simvastatin to 80 mg OD, or an alternative statin of similar efficacy and cost

Table 3.2 Doses of commonly used statins and reduction in low–density lipoprotein (LDL) cholesterol

Drug	Dose (mg/day)	% LDL cholesterol reduction
Atorvastatin	10	39
Pravastatin	40	34
Simvastatin	20–40	35–41
Fluvastatin	40–80	25–35
Rosuvastatin	5–10	39–45

may be considered if the targets are not achieved. Further LDL cholesterol reduction may also be achieved with the addition of ezetimibe, which inhibits the absorption of dietary and biliary cholesterol (Figure 3.1).

Unlike the effect on LDL cholesterol, the effect of statins on triglycerides and HDL cholesterol are less impressive. Current data suggest that triglycerides and HDL cholesterol may be considered targets for treatment following lowering of LDL cholesterol in high-risk patients. Treatment options include fibrates, nicotinic acid and fish oils. Aggressive glycaemic control may lower serum triglycerides and other causes of hypertriglycidaemia should be excluded (e.g. renal impairment or liver, particularly alcohol-related disease).

A meta-analysis of 53 trials using fibrates and 30 trials using nicotinic acid reported a 25% and 27% reduction in major coronary events respectively. A fibrate (particularly fenofibrate) has been recommended as first-line treatment of hypertriglycidaemia

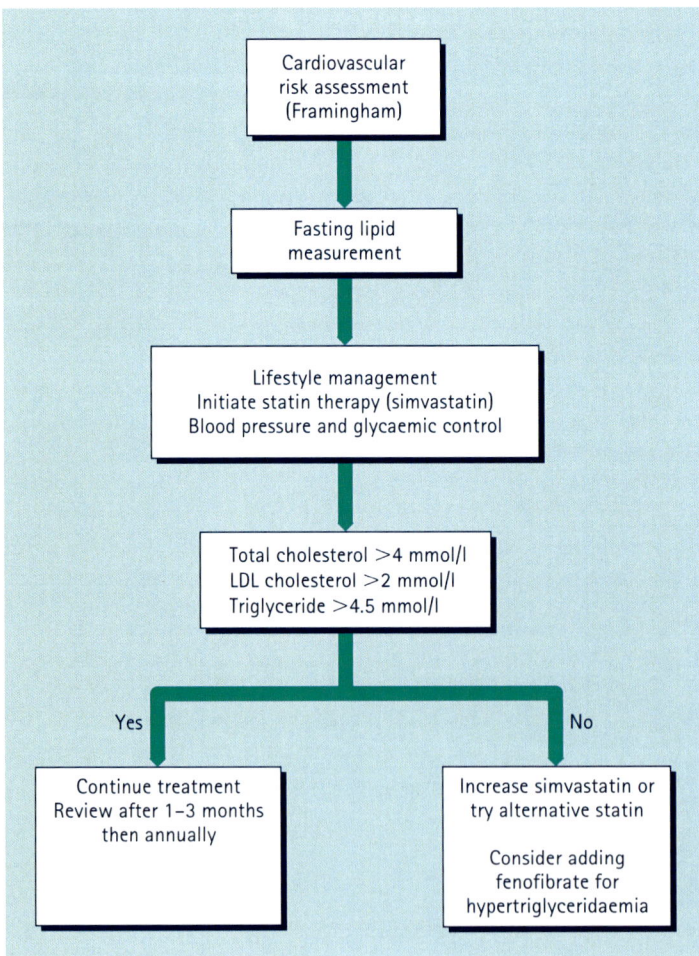

Figure 3.1 Treatment of dyslipidaemia. LDL, low-density lipoprotein.

(triglyceride >4.5 mmol/l) after treatment of other potential causes. In some cases of persistent dyslipidaemia despite intensification of statin therapy, combination treatment should be considered. Combining statins with fibrates or niacin offers significant reductions in triglycerides and increases in HDL cholesterol. The combined use of fibrates and statins has been limited by concerns over myositis and rhabdomyolysis. However, recent pharmacokinetic studies indicate that fenofibrate, unlike gemfibrozil, do not increase blood levels of statins and, therefore, may be safe to use in combination therapy.

The combination of niacin and statin probably does not increase the risk of myositis or rhabdomyolysis, but niacin does appear to worsen glycaemic control, albeit correctable with titration of antihyperglycaemic medications. Hence, treatment with niacin should generally be managed by lipid specialists. Combination therapy with statins and fish oils also offers additional triglyceride lowering compared with statin therapy alone, although increases in HDL cholesterol levels usually will not match those seen with fibrates or niacin. The indications and contraindications of different classes of lipid-lowering therapy are listed in Table 3.3.

Recent Developments

Rimonabant, a selective endocannabinoid receptor antagonist, generated considerable interest as multi-centre trials (the RIO studies) confirmed the efficacy of rimonabant in reducing body weight (sustained for up to 2 years) compared to placebo, which was associated with significant improvements in HDL cholesterol, triglycerides and glycaemic control (in patients with diabetes). Despite these promising results, the associated adverse psychiatric effects of anxiety and depression have led to its withdrawal.

Table 3.3 Indications and contraindications for different classes of lipid–lowering drugs

Drugs‡	Indications	Caution	Contraindications
HMG-CoA reductase inhibitor (statins)	Atherosclerotic vascular disease Raised cardiovascular risk Hypercholesterolaemia	Renal impairment Concurrent use of drugs metabolized via P450	Avoid with gemfibrozil Significant liver disease Previous myositis with statins
Fibrates	Type III hyperlipoproteinaemia Hypertriglyceridaemia	Renal failure Concurrent statin therapy†	Gemfibrozil with statin
Nicotinic acid	Hypertriglyceridaemia Mixed hyperlipidaemia (low high-density lipoprotein cholesterol)	Renal failure Liver disease Diabetes (worsen glycaemic control)	Diarrhoea or flushing (may worsen symtoms)
Fish oils (ω-3-acid ethyl esters)	Hypertriglyceridaemia Post-myocardial infarction	Haemorrhagic disorders Aspirin-sensitive asthma	None

†Some statins are metabolized via the P450 pathway (e.g. atorvastatin and simvastatin). Other drugs metabolized via this pathway may interact with these statins (e.g. ciclosporin, antifungals and amiodarone). Expert advice should be sought.
‡Fibrates, nicotinic acid and anion exchange resins (not listed) should not be used routinely in the setting of primary prevention.

The recent JUPITER trial has also challenged conventional cholesterol-based risk factor management. This large study included patients with satisfactory cholesterol levels but raised highly-sensitive C-reactive protein levels, and demonstrated significant reduction in cardiovascular events with rosuvastatin in these patients compared to placebo. The highly-sensitive CRP however, is not yet widely available. Nonetheless, this study has generated considerable debates with potential expansion of the indications for statin therapy in the prevention of cardiovascular events.

Modified-release niacin has also generated significant interests as an add-on to statin therapy. The ARBITER 6-HALTS trial compared niacin and ezetimibe in patients already on statins with carotid intima-media thickness (CIMT) as the surrogate endpoint. The addition of niacin resulted in regression of CIMT, but there were no significant changes with ezetimibe.

Conclusion

Treatment of total and LDL cholesterol is the primary aim of lipid treatment. This may be achieved in the majority of cases with the use of statins (simvastatin 40 mg OD is recommended for primary prevention of cardiovascular events by current NICE guidance). However, residual cardiovascular risk remains high even when LDL cholesterol is treated to target levels. The treatment of dyslipidaemia should therefore be considered. Combining statins with fenofibrate or niacin offers significant reductions in triglycerides and increases in HDL cholesterol. Referral to specialist lipid clinics should be considered.

Further Reading

Grundy SM, Cleeman JI, Merz CN, *et al*; Coordinating Committee of the National Cholesterol Education Program; National Heart, Lung, and Blood Institute; American College of Cardiology Foundation; American Heart Association. Implications of recent clinical trials for the National Cholesterol Education Program Adult Treatment Panel III guidelines. *Arterioscler Thromb Vasc Biol* 2004; **24**: e149–61.

National Institute of Clinical Excellence. The management of type-2 diabetes. May 2008.

Ridker PM, Danielson E, Fonseca FA, *et al*. Rosuvastatin to prevent vascular events in men and women with elevated C-reactive protein. *N Engl J Med* 2008; **359**: 2195–207.

SECTION TWO

02

Coronary Artery Disease

4	Assessment of stable angina
5	Treatment of stable angina
6	Management of acute coronary syndrome
7	Initial management of ST elevation myocardial infarction
8	Hypotension in acute myocardial infarction
9	Cardiogenic shock
10	Peri-infarct arrhythmia
11	Secondary prevention (lifestyle, risk factors and drug treatment)

PROBLEM

4 Assessment of stable angina

Case History

Over the last 8 weeks, a 68-year-old man has noticed a mild dull ache in his chest and left arm occurring while out walking his dog. It occurs predictably on walking up a steep hill, resolving after a few minutes on resting. He has never had chest pain at rest and he manages all his normal daily activities. He is a smoker (30 pack-years) and is on bendroflumethiazide for hypertension.

What is the diagnosis and what is the likely cause?

How should this patient be managed?

What is the classification of symptom severity?

What initial investigations would you undertake?

How would you confirm the diagnosis of coronary artery disease and risk stratify the patient?

This patient's presentation is consistent with stable angina pectoris.

Background

 Stable angina is caused by an imbalance between the supply and demand for oxygenated blood to the myocardium. The commonest cause is obstructive coronary artery disease. Other causes are listed in Table 4.1.

Table 4.1 Causes of angina

Cardiac
    Hypertrophic cardiomyopathy
    Aortic stenosis
    Hypertensive heart disease with left ventricular hypertrophy
    Severe pulmonary hypertension with right ventricular hypertrophy

Vascular
    Coronary artery spasm
    Microvascular disease (cardiological syndrome 'X')

Non-cardiac
    Thyrotoxicosis
    Severe anaemia

How should this patient be managed?

A careful history and examination should be undertaken to clarify the patient's symptoms, to help to identify any non-coronary artery disease causes of angina and to identify risk factors (Table 4.2).

Table 4.2 Risk factors of coronary artery disease

- Male sex
- Increasing age
- Smoking
- Increased body mass index
- Sedentary lifestyle
- Diabetes mellitus
- Hypertension
- Hyperlipidaemia

What is the classification of symptom severity?

The Canadian Cardiovascular Society classification is the most commonly used to assess symptom severity. It classes symptoms from class I–IV, as described in Table 4.3. This man's symptoms equate to Canadian Cardiovascular Society class I.

What initial investigations would you undertake?

Initial investigations include full blood count, renal function, fasting blood glucose, lipid profile, thyroid function tests, an electrocardiogram (ECG) and echocardiogram. A normal ECG does not exclude coronary artery disease, although the presence of Q waves or

04 Assessment of stable angina

Table 4.3 Canadian Cardiovascular Society (CCS) classification

CCS class	Symptoms
Class I	Angina only occurs with extraordinary exertion at work or recreation with ordinary activities not resulting in symptoms
Class II	Ordinary activity slightly limited by symptoms such as walking more than two blocks on a level surface or climbing more than one flight of stairs at a normal pace
Class III	Symptoms result in marked limitation of ordinary physical activity, such as walking one to two blocks on a level surface or climbing one flight of stairs at normal pace
Class IV	Chest discomfort occurs at minimal activity or stress or at rest

persistent ST segment depression may indicate the diagnosis of coronary artery disease and are associated with an unfavourable outcome. In addition, electrocardiographic evidence of left ventricular hypertrophy may indicate hypertensive heart disease or aortic stenosis. Left bundle branch block may indicate previous myocardial injury or left ventricular dysfunction. Echocardiography may show regional wall motion abnormalities, which may be indicative of coronary artery disease, and may also identify non-coronary causes of angina, such as hypertrophic cardiomyopathy or severe aortic stenosis (Figure 4.1).

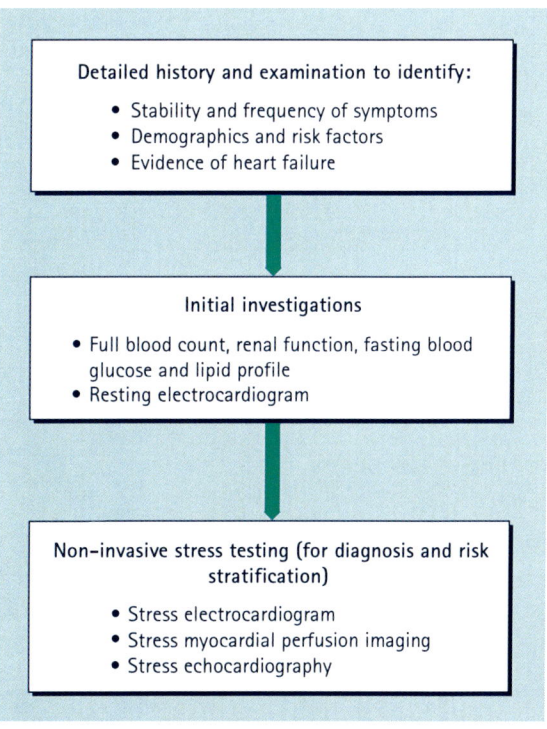

Figure 4.1 Initial assessment of a patient with chronic stable angina.

How would you confirm the diagnosis of coronary artery disease and risk stratify the patient?

Non-invasive methods of assessing myocardial ischaemia involve:

- applying a stress to the myocardium (increase oxygen consumption) to provoke ischaemia, or produce coronary vasodilatation;
- followed by an assessment of the resulting ischaemia.

Methods of inducing myocardial ischaemia

The most useful and physiological method of inducing ischaemia is through exercise. However, a significant proportion of patients may be unable to exercise (e.g. osteoarthritis) and pharmacological methods may be used instead. Exercise stress testing is generally more sensitive and specific in males compared with females. An exercise test is considered adequate if the patient achieves 85% or more of an age-adjusted maximum heart rate per minute (220 minus age). Contraindications to exercise stress testing are outlined below.

- Uncontrolled hypertension (>200 mmHg systolic and/or >110 mmHg diastolic).
- Left bundle branch block on the baseline ECG or a paced rhythm.
- Suspected unstable angina or acute myocardial infarction.
- Acute myocarditis or pericarditis.
- Symptomatic severe aortic stenosis.
- Uncontrolled, symptomatic heart failure.
- Uncontrolled arrhythmia.
- Inability to perform an exercise ECG due to comorbidity or disability.

Pharmacological methods include the use of adenosine, dipyridamole or dobutamine. Adenosine causes coronary microvascular vasodilatation resulting in a discrepancy in myocardial blood flow with increased perfusion in areas of the myocardium supplied by normal arteries and relatively less perfusion in areas supplied by stenosed vessels. Dipyridamole also causes coronary microvascular vasodilatation by inhibiting the cellular uptake of adenosine. However, due to its mechanism of action, its onset is slower and is of longer duration. Dobutamine is a β_1 agonist and, at low doses, has a positive inotropic effect. Higher doses produce an additional chronotropic effect resulting in an increase in heart rate. The plasma half-life is 2–3 minutes. Similar to exercise, an adequate test is considered to have been achieved if the heart rate increases to 85% or more of the maximum age predicted heart rate. If this is not achieved, despite maximal doses of dobutamine, intravenous atropine can be given.

Methods of assessing myocardial ischaemia

Twelve-lead electrocardiogram

A continuously recorded 12-lead ECG during the stress can indicate the presence of ischaemia. A test is considered positive if the patient develops 1-mm ST segment depression in the context of chest pain or 2-mm ST segment depression in the absence of chest pain. Features that indicate high risk of future cardiac events include:

- Early positive tests (<3 minutes of the standard Bruce protocol).
- A strongly positive test (>2 mm ST segment depression) with sustained ST segment depression after exercise cessation (>3 minutes).

- Ischaemia at low heart rate (<120 beats/minute).
- Blunted blood pressure response to exercise or drop in blood pressure at peak exercise.
- Significant ventricular arrhythmias at low work load (<120 beats/minute).
- Inability to complete two stages of the standard Bruce protocol (<6 minutes).

The stress test should be terminated when ischaemia is demonstrated. Other reasons for terminating the stress test include significant arrhythmia, blood pressure drop, symptoms of light-headedness and if the patient is unable to continue.

In the absence of contraindications, this patient underwent exercise testing, which demonstrated ECG changes suggestive of ischaemia after 9 minutes.

Echocardiography

Echocardiography, undertaken continuously during application of a stress, allows an assessment of reversible myocardial ischaemia, viability and the presence of scar (Table 4.4). Areas of myocardium supplied by stenosed vessels exhibit normal wall motion at rest but become impaired with stress. Stress echocardiography is limited by patients with poor echocardiographic images (e.g. obese patients).

Table 4.4 Interpretation of wall motion in response to stress

Interpretation	Baseline	Low-level stress	Peak and post-stress function
Normal	Normal	Normal or hyperdynamic response	Hyperdynamic response
Ischaemia	Normal	Normal or in the context of severe coronary artery disease can deteriorate	Deterioration
Viable and ischaemic	Resting regional wall abnormality	Improved motion	Deterioration
Scar tissue	Resting regional wall abnormality (usually akinetic)	No change	No change

Patients may be risk stratified based on the findings of the stress echocardiographic study (Table 4.5).

Table 4.5 Risk stratification with stress echocardiography

Finding on stress echocardiography	Degree of risk
Extensive ischaemia with wall motion abnormality involving >2 segments developing at low dose of dobutamine (<10 mg/kg/min) or at a low heart rate (<120 beats/min)	High (annual cardiovascular mortality of >3%)
Mild/moderate resting left ventricular dysfunction (left ventricular ejection fraction 35–49%) Limited ischaemia with a wall motion abnormality involving <2 segments only at higher doses of dobutamine	Moderate (annual cardiovascular mortality of 1–3%)
Normal wall motion or no change of limited resting wall motion abnormalities during stress	Low (annual cardiovascular mortality of <1%)

Radionuclide scintigraphy

This imaging modality involves single photon emission computed tomography (SPECT) utilizing radio-pharmaceuticals such as thallium 201 or technetium 99^m (Figure 4.2 – *see inside front cover*). With thallium, relative myocardial ischaemia is demonstrated by differences in the distribution of the thallium, whereas with technetium, two injections of the radio-isotope are given and a comparison is made between uptake in the resting and stress images. Reversible defects indicate reversible myocardial ischaemia with fixed defects indicating previous myocardial infarction. In comparison with normal scans, patients who have abnormal perfusion defects are at 15-fold higher risk of mortality from cardiovascular causes. The greatest risk is associated with those with multiple segments of abnormal perfusion or large defects, particularly involving the anterior wall. The proximal septum correlates to a proximal left anterior descending artery stenosis and reversible ischaemia in this segment additionally indicates poor prognosis. Increased lung uptake and dilatation of the left ventricle are markers of severe coronary artery disease. Contraindications to stress imaging are outlined in Table 4.6.

Developments that are more recent include the use of cardiac magnetic resonance imaging (MRI) with stress testing. The use of gadolinium enhancement with stress testing may identify areas of ischaemia. Although images may be superior to echocardiographic studies, cardiac MRI may be limited by claustrophobia. CT angiography has been advancing rapidly over the last few years and may provide reliable non-invasive assessment of coronary anatomy and stenoses. However, CT angiography is not widely available.

The gold standard for determining the presence of coronary artery stenoses is coronary angiography; however, due to the risk involved (on average a 1 in 1000 risk of a serious complication, e.g. myocardial infarction or stroke) this imaging modality is reserved for the following patients:

- Inadequate control of symptoms despite optimal medical treatment.
- Those patients who have high-risk features on stress testing.
- Moderate or severe left ventricular systolic impairment.
- Those requiring major surgical intervention.

The demonstration of coronary artery disease is associated with an increased risk of future cardiac events. Stenoses >70% are sufficient to limit flow and result in myocardial ischaemia. However, the severity of stenosis does not predict plaque stability and 60% of patients who develop an acute myocardial infarction have a 50% or less diameter stenosis at the site of occurrence of plaque rupture resulting in the myocardial infarction. Hence,

Table 4.6 Contraindications to stress imaging

- Uncontrolled hypertension (>200 mmHg systolic and/or >110 mmHg diastolic)
- Suspected unstable angina or acute myocardial infarction
- Acute myocarditis or pericarditis
- Uncontrolled, symptomatic heart failure
- Symptomatic severe aortic stenosis

treatment of significant stenoses may not necessarily reduce the risk of future acute coronary syndrome.

Recent Developments

CT angiography has undergone considerable advances over the last few years and now provides anatomical characterization of coronary artery disease almost comparable with invasive coronary angiography. Indeed, CT angiography is now routinely available in a number of centres. Cardiac MRI, coupled with a pharmacological stress protocol provides greater resolution compared with radionuclide studies and provides functional assessment of myocardial ischaemia. Non-invasive assessment of coronary artery disease will continue to evolve with advances in imaging technology.

Conclusion

Assessment of chest pain suggestive of ischaemia, described as angina pectoris, should begin with careful history and examination. While obstructive coronary artery disease is the most common cause of angina pectoris, it is not invariably so and other causes should be excluded. Non-invasive assessment with stress testing allows risk stratification and guide therapy, and should be considered before invasive assessment of coronary artery disease.

Further Reading

Fraker TD Jr, Fihn SD; 2002 Chronic Stable Angina Writing Committee; American College of Cardiology; American Heart Association, Gibbons RJ, Abrams J, Chatterjee K, *et al.* 2007 chronic angina focused update of the ACC/AHA 2002 guidelines for the management of patients with chronic stable angina: a report of the American College of Cardiology/American Heart Association Task Force on Practice Guidelines Writing Group to develop the focused update of the 2002 guidelines for the management of patients with chronic stable angina. *J Am Coll Cardiol* 2007; **50**: 2264–74.

§02 Coronary Artery Disease

PROBLEM

05 Treatment of stable angina

Case History

A 65-year-old patient attended the Rapid Access Angina Clinic with symptoms of angina that had occurred while running on a treadmill at his local gymnasium. He has a history of hypertension on a thiazide diuretic, but no known diabetes. He is an ex-smoker. His resting heart rate was 76 beats/minute and blood pressure was 142/88 mmHg. He underwent an exercise stress test during which he managed 6.5 minutes of the standard Bruce Protocol with appropriate blood pressure response and achieved a maximum heart rate of 137 beats/minute, which represented 85% of his maximum age predicted heart rate, before developing chest pain with 1-mm horizontal ST segment depression in the lateral leads.

What are the treatment options available to this patient?

Despite medical therapy he continues to be symptomatic, how would you manage him?

Background

This patient has stable coronary artery disease. Treatment is directed at improving quality of life by reducing symptoms and the risk of future cardiovascular morbidity and mortality. Medical therapy, percutaneous transluminal coronary angioplasty (PTCA) and coronary artery bypass graft surgery (CABG) have all been shown to improve symptoms, but only medical therapy and CABG have been shown to improve prognosis. This patient can be considered low risk on the basis of his stress test and, therefore, should be managed medically, in addition to risk factor modification (Figure 5.1).

Pharmacological treatment

Antiplatelet agents

All patients with cardiovascular disease should be treated with aspirin 75 mg OD. This has been shown to reduce the risk of myocardial infarction and cardiovascular death by about 25% in patients with stable angina. Clopidogrel 75 mg OD has been shown to be at least as effective as aspirin and is a reasonable alternative in patients with genuine aspirin intolerance. Combined aspirin and clopidogrel may have additional benefit in patients at high risk (e.g. established cardiovascular disease) but at the expense of increased bleeding complications.

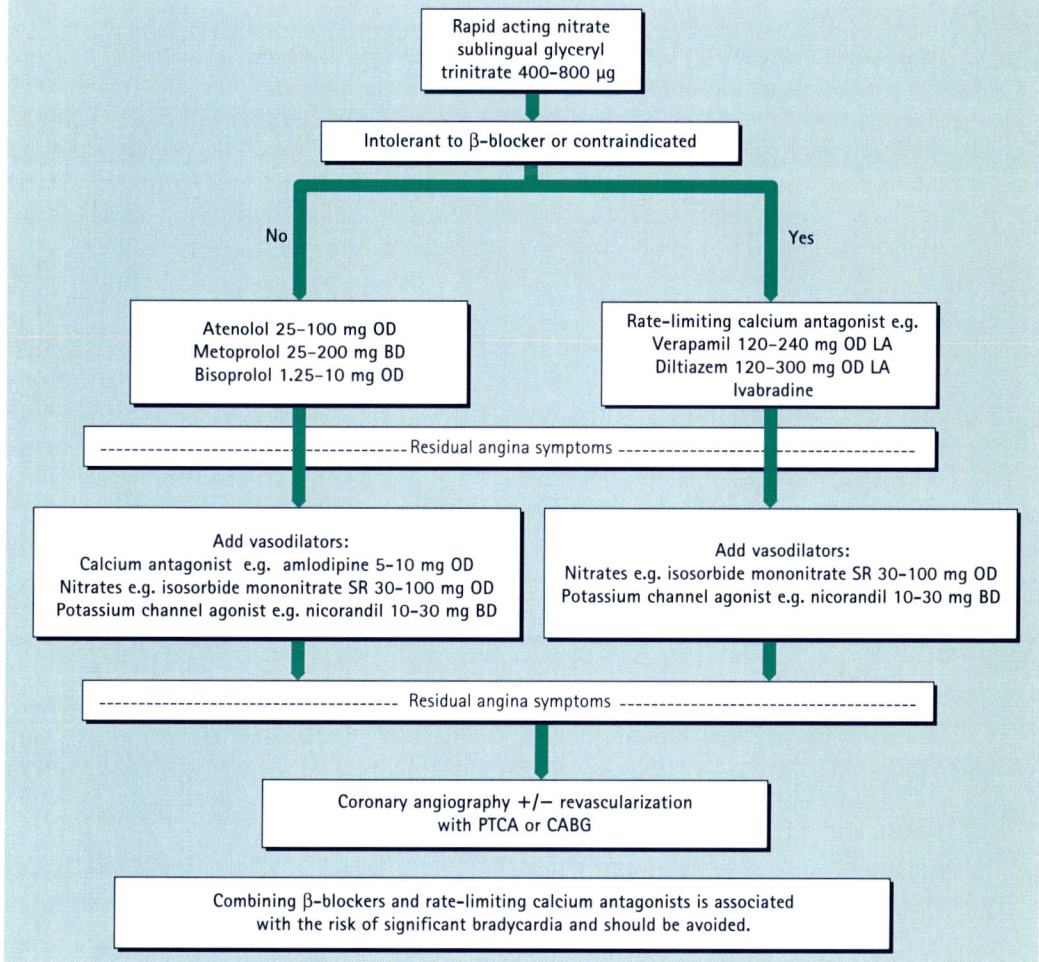

Figure 5.1 Anti-anginal treatment of chronic stable angina. BD, twice daily; CABG, coronary artery bypass graft surgery; LA, long-acting; OD, once daily; PTCA, percutaneous transluminal coronary angioplasty; SR, slow-release.

Anti-anginal medication (Figure 5.1)

Medical treatment for angina can generally be divided into two groups based on their dominant mechanism of action: rate-lowering agents and vasodilators. The effect of different anti-anginal therapy may therefore be complementary.

Beta-blockers

This group of drugs blocks the β_1 adrenergic receptor resulting in a reduction in heart rate, force of contraction of the myocardium and, hence, reduces cardiac work and oxygen demand. This is believed to be the mechanism for the effective relief of anginal symptoms. The dose of the β-blocker should be titrated as tolerated to achieve a resting heart rate of between 50 and 60 beats/minute. Although no prognostic benefit has been shown in stable angina, β-blockers have been shown to improve prognosis following a myocardial infarction. β-blockers may exacerbate bronchospasm, especially in patients with asthma.

Calcium channel blockers

Dihydropyridine calcium antagonists, such as amlodipine and nifedipine, act as vasodilators with no negative chronotropic effect on the heart. Conversely, the non-dihydropyridine calcium antagonists, such as verapamil and diltiazem, reduce heart rate, are negatively inotropic and cause less vasodilatation. Both groups reduce symptoms but they have not been shown to reduce the risk of myocardial infarction or improve mortality. Short-acting preparations of nifedipine should be avoided. Dihydropyridine calcium antagonists may cause peripheral oedema and verapamil may cause constipation.

Nitrates

Nitrates reduce left ventricular preload and afterload and are coronary artery vasodilators, which are believed to be the dominant mechanism of action in reducing myocardial ischaemia. They alleviate symptoms, and increase effort tolerance, but have not been shown to improve cardiovascular morbidity and mortality. Sublingual preparations allow a rapid onset of action but have a short duration of action. Longer-acting oral preparations, or transdermal patches, are also available but require an 8-hour 'nitrate-free' period to prevent the development of tolerance. Headaches, flushing and light-headedness are the most common side effects.

Potassium channel agonists

Potassium channel agonists, e.g. nicorandil, cause vasodilatation and have a potentially cardioprotective effect. The IONA study (Impact of Nicorandil in Angina) showed significant reduction in clinical events with the use of nicorandil 20 mg twice daily. Nicorandil may cause headaches.

Ivabradine

Ivabradine is a selective I_f channel blocker. The I_f channel current is responsible for the pacemaker current in the sinoatrial node. Ivabradine, by slowing sinoatrial node discharge, slows the heart rate and thereby reduces symptoms of angina. A post hoc sub-analysis of the BEAUTIFUL (morbidity mortality evaluation of the If inhibitor ivabradine in patients with coronary disease and left ventricular dysfunction) trial suggest reduction in rates of hospitalisatons for fatal and non-fatal myocardial infarction in patients with limiting angina. The effect of ivabradine on cardiovascular outcomes will be evaluated in future studies.

Ranolazine

Ranolazine has been shown to improve exercise duration in patients with angina without significant effect on heart rate and blood pressure. The mechanism of action is unclear. Proposed mechanisms include partial inhibition of fatty acid oxidation (by improving metabolic efficiency) and inhibition of late sodium channel (preventing calcium overload). Despite improvements in exercise duration in patients with angina, there was no significant reduction in cardiovascular events in the MERLIN (Metabolic Efficiency with Ranolazine for Less Ischaemia in Non-ST elevation myocardial infarction) TIMI-36 trial of 6560 patients with non-ST elevation myocardial infarction. Of note, patients treated with ranolazine had a lower incidence of arrhythmias (although there was a small increase in QT interval) and a mild reduction in HbA1c.

05 Treatment of stable angina

Angiotensin-converting enzyme inhibitors
Angiotensin-converting enzyme inhibitors reduce both preload and afterload and, hence, reduce myocardial oxygen demand. The HOPE study (Heart Outcomes Prevention Evaluation) showed treatment with ramipril resulted in a 16% reduction in all-cause mortality, myocardial infarction and stroke in patients with cardiovascular disease (55% had chronic stable angina). The EUROPA trial (EUropean trial on Reduction Of cardiac events with Perindopril in stable coronary Artery disease) showed similar benefits with perindopril.

Lipid-lowering medication
Lipid-lowering treatment is associated with a significant reduction in cardiovascular events and disease progression. The Joint British Society guidelines for secondary prevention, in patients with established coronary artery disease, recommend a total cholesterol level of <4 mmol/l with a low-density lipoprotein cholesterol level <2 mmol/l. First-line treatment is a HMG-CoA inhibitor (statin) and all patients with established coronary artery disease, irrespective of their cholesterol level, should be treated with a statin (e.g. simvastatin 40 mg OD). Statins may cause muscle aches, minor increases in creatinine kinase and liver function tests and, rarely, rhabdomyolysis.

This patient was commenced on aspirin, metoprolol, ramipril and simvastatin.

Despite medical therapy he continues to be symptomatic, how would you manage him?

Patients who continue to have angina symptoms, despite optimization of medical treatment and risk factor modification, should be considered for coronary artery revascularization. The choice of whether this is undertaken by PTCA or CABG surgery is dictated by the severity and extent of the patient's coronary artery stenoses (Figure 5.2).

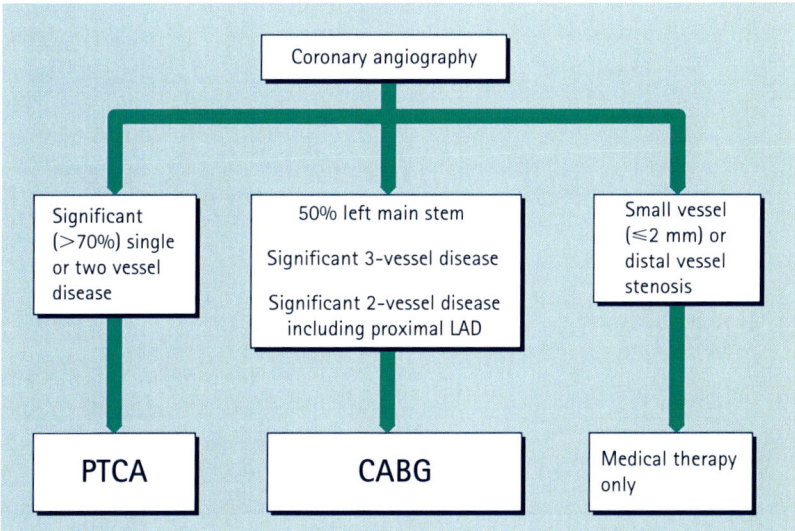

Figure 5.2 Recommended treatment following coronary angiography. CABG, coronary artery bypass graft surgery; LAD, left anterior descending; PTCA, percutaneous transluminal coronary angioplasty.

Percutaneous transluminal coronary angioplasty and stenting

Although PTCA has not been shown to improve survival in stable angina, it is an effective treatment for improving symptoms of angina, which often results in a reduction in the number of different anti-anginal medications, improvement in effort tolerance and quality of life. However, the risks of the procedure (risk of myocardial infarction, stroke or death – depending on the complexity of coronary stenoses, generally <1%) should be balanced with the potential benefit. It is also the preferred mode of revascularization in patients with severe comorbidity (e.g. chronic obstructive pulmonary disease) that makes the risk of surgery prohibitive.

Coronary angioplasty and stenting may be complicated by restenosis. The need for repeat angioplasty procedures may be higher than 15% depending on the type of stent used, patient characteristics and complexity of the coronary disease. The introduction of drug-eluting stents have reduced this risk but concerns about late stent thrombosis resulting in myocardial infarction and death have emerged recently and remain a subject of considerable debate and controversy.

Coronary artery bypass graft surgery

As with medical treatment, CABG surgery significantly improves the symptoms of angina with the reduction in the need for anti-anginal medication and improved effort tolerance. However, in comparison with medical treatment, CABG surgery improves long-term survival in patients with stable angina when the coronary artery disease is sufficiently severe. Previous studies have demonstrated improvement in cardiovascular morbidity and mortality with CABG surgery in patients with high-risk coronary artery disease: a 50% or more left main stem coronary artery stenosis, three-vessel disease or two-vessel disease, including a severe proximal left anterior descending artery stenosis. Prognostic benefit is also seen in patients with impaired left ventricular systolic function and those with diabetes mellitus. It is also preferred in those with concomitant valvular, aortic root or congenital heart disease that will require surgery. Long-term graft patency depends on whether venous or arterial grafts are used. After 5 years, 20% of venous grafts have become non-functional and this percentage has risen to 50% after 10 years. This is in contrast to internal mammary artery grafts where 90% are still patent at 10 years.

Studies to date comparing CABG with PTCA suggest a lower rate of recurrence of symptoms with surgical intervention in addition to lower rates of reintervention. The development of drug-eluting stents, which reduce the risk of restenosis with PTCA and stenting, has prompted ongoing randomized studies comparing surgery and stenting.

Recent Developments

The recent COURAGE (Clinical Outcomes Utilizing Revascularization and Aggressive Drug Evaluation) trial compared contemporary medical treatment with and without invasive revascularization (percutaneous coronary intervention [PCI]) in patients with stable coronary artery disease. Patients with persistent class IV symptoms or a markedly positive stress test were excluded. Over 4.6 years, there was no significant difference in death and myocardial infarction between the two groups. Although PCI was associated with an initially better quality of life and symptoms, this difference was no longer significant by 36 months. Of note, almost 33% of patients initially randomized to medical treatment alone underwent revascularization. Hence, in the absence of high-risk features from non-invasive testing or persistent severe angina, medical treatment without revascularization may be a reasonable initial treatment strategy.

Conclusion

Medical treatment is a reasonable first-line therapy for patients with stable coronary artery disease in the absence of high-risk features on non-invasive stress testing. Coronary revascularization may be considered in patients with persistent symptoms despite medical treatment. Both percutaneous coronary intervention (with stenting) and CABG surgery are effective symptomatic treatment but only the latter has been shown to provide additional prognostic benefit over medical treatment alone in some patients with high-risk coronary artery disease.

Further Reading

Boden WE, O'Rourke RA, Teo KK, *et al.* Optimal medical therapy with or without PCI for stable coronary disease. *N Engl J Med* 2007; **356**: 1503–16.

Fraker TD Jr, Fihn SD; 2002 Chronic Stable Angina Writing Committee; American College of Cardiology; American Heart Association, Gibbons RJ, Abrams J, Chatterjee K, *et al.* Chronic angina focused update of the ACC/AHA 2002 guidelines for the management of patients with chronic stable angina: a report of the American College of Cardiology/American Heart Association Task Force on Practice Guidelines Writing Group to develop the focused update of the 2002 guidelines for the management of patients with chronic stable angina. *J Am Coll Cardiol* 2007; **50**: 2264–74.

PROBLEM

06 Management of acute coronary syndrome

Case History

A 66-year-old woman presented with three episodes of central chest pain associated with sweating and breathlessness over the last 24 hours. These chest pains occurred at rest and minimal exertion, lasting over 30 minutes. She had a body mass index of 34 kg/m² and was hypertensive. Her regular medications include aspirin, simvastatin and amlodipine. She is a smoker of 10 cigarettes a day. At presentation, she was free of chest pain having been treated with analgesia with a blood pressure of 142/78 mmHg and heart rate of

80 beats/minute. Her electrocardiogram (ECG) is shown in Figure 6.1. Her 12-hour troponin T was 0.8 µg/l.

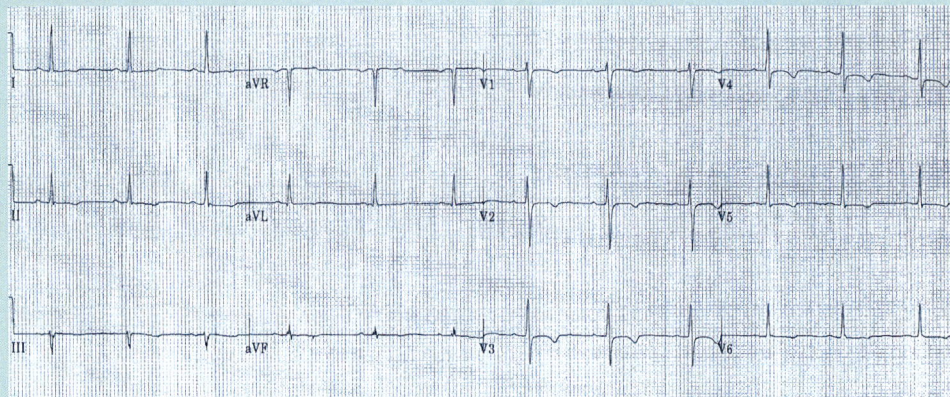

Figure 6.1 Electrocardiogram.

What does her ECG show and what is the diagnosis?

How would you risk-stratify this patient?

How would you define this patient's risk based on her ECG changes?

Would you risk-stratify this woman as low, medium or high risk based on troponin?

How would you manage this patient?

The patient's ECG shows sinus rhythm with anterolateral T wave inversion. In the context of her presentation, these ECG changes indicate myocardial ischaemia.

Background

This patient has an acute coronary syndrome defined more accurately as a non-ST elevation myocardial infarction (NSTEMI) (Figure 6.2). The acute clinical presentation contrasts with that of stable coronary disease. An acute coronary syndrome is a spectrum of clinical presentation of the same disease process and can be divided into:

1 unstable angina, which is acute (generally <1 week) development or abrupt worsening of symptoms);
2 NSTEMI; and
3 ST elevation myocardial infarction (STEMI).

The extent of haemorrhage into an atheromatous plaque, thrombus formation, coronary artery vasoconstriction and consequent reduction in coronary blood flow determines the clinical syndrome that ensues.

The management of acute coronary syndromes varies depending on the clinical presentation. Unlike STEMI, unstable angina and NSTEMI do not require immediate reper-

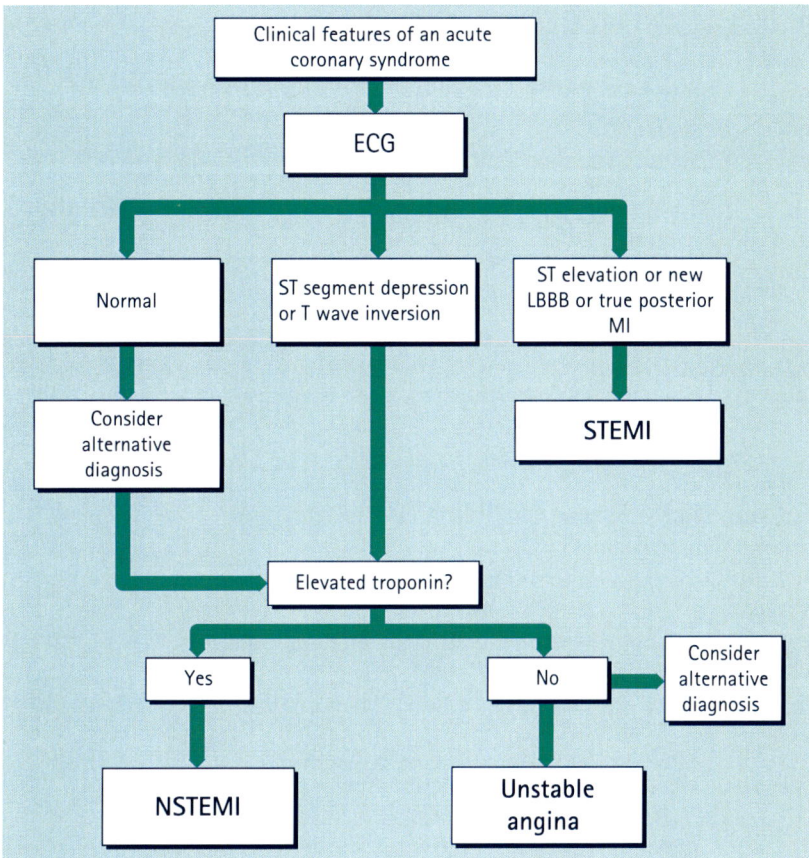

Figure 6.2 Algorithm for defining type of acute coronary syndrome. LBBB, left bundle branch block; MI, myocardial infarction; NSTEMI, non-ST elevation myocardial infarction; STEMI, ST elevation myocardial infarction.

fusion therapy. The distinction between unstable angina and NSTEMI is based on elevated cardiac enzymes. The current definition of myocardial infarction is based on elevation in cardiac enzymes, particularly troponin, which is a highly selective cardiac protein, should be taken as evidence of myocardial necrosis and, hence, a myocardial infarction. The troponin should be measured on admission and at 12 hours since the last episode of chest pain. Of note, the absence of troponin elevation excludes myocardial infarction, but it does not exclude an acute coronary syndrome (unstable angina).

How would you risk-stratify this patient?

A number of scoring systems have been developed to help risk-stratify patients presenting with an acute coronary syndrome. The most commonly used is the TIMI (Thrombolysis in Myocardial Infarction) Risk Score that was derived from trials of low molecular weight heparins. Other scoring systems, while more accurate, tend to be more complex and less clinically practical (e.g. the GRACE [Global Registry of Acute Coronary Events] score).

Table 6.1 Thrombolysis in Myocardial Infarction Risk Score 14-day event rate

Risk	Number of risk factors	14-day event rate (%)
Low	0/1	4.7
	2	8.3
Medium	3	13.2
	4	19.9
High	5	26.2
	6/7	40.9

The TIMI system assigns a binary score (0 or 1) to the seven independent risk factors with similar predictive value; the higher the score the higher the risk of death or recurrent ischaemia at 14 days (Table 6.1). The seven risk factors include:

1. Sixty-five years of age or older.
2. Three or more risk factors for coronary artery disease (including diabetes mellitus, smoking, family history of ischaemic heart disease, hypertension and hypercholesterolaemia).
3. Significant coronary artery stenoses.
4. ST segment deviation.
5. Two or more anginal episodes within the previous 24 hours.
6. The use of aspirin prior to admission.
7. Elevated cardiac markers (creatine kinase or troponin).

This patient is therefore at high risk based on age, aspirin use, elevated troponin, ECG changes and recurrent chest pain (TIMI risk score of 5).

How would you define this patient's risk based on her ECG changes?

This patient has deep symmetrical T wave inversion on her ECG, which would define her as high risk of future cardiac events (Table 6.2).

Table 6.2 Risk stratification from ECG

Low-risk ECG	Normal ECG or with T-wave flattening or <1 mm T wave inversion
Medium-risk ECG	T-wave inversion of >1 mm or ST segment depression of 1 mm or less
High-risk ECG	Deep symmetrical T-wave inversion or >1 mm ST segment depression or transient ST segment elevation

Would you risk-stratify this woman as low, medium or high risk based on troponin?

Troponin I and T are highly specific to the myocardium and relate to structural proteins, which are involved in the binding of calcium during myocyte contraction. They are released into the blood following tissue necrosis reaching peak levels at 12 hours and remain elevated for 7 days. There is a direct correlation between troponin level and risk of death. The higher the troponin the greater the 5-month risk of death and myocardial infarction as determined in the FRISC study (Fragmin during Instability in Coronary Artery Disease; peak troponin in the first 24 hours post-enrolment). This patient is considered high risk based on her troponin levels (Table 6.3).

06 Management of acute coronary syndrome

Table 6.3 Risk assessment based on troponin level (FRISC study)

Risk	Serum troponin T	Risk of death or myocardial infarction at 5 months (%)
Low	<0.06 µg/l	4.3
Medium	0.06–0.59 µg/l	10.5
High	>0.6 µg/l	16.1

How would you manage this patient? (Figure 6.3)

1. The patient should receive bed rest with continuous ECG monitoring and pulse oximetry with inhaled oxygen therapy. In addition to these supportive treatments, patients with NSTEMI should be treated with antiplatelet agents, antithrombotic therapy, anti-anginal therapy and coronary revascularization. Patients not on lipid-lowering therapy should also be commenced on a statin, as some data suggest better clinical outcome with early aggressive statin treatment.

2. *Antiplatelet therapy.* All patients should be treated with 300 mg of aspirin (loading dose) and, thereafter, 75 mg OD. This has been shown to reduce death or myocardial infarction by 50% as compared with placebo. In addition, all patients, unless contraindicated, should receive 300 mg of clopidogrel (loading dose) followed by 75 mg OD thereafter. In the CURE (Clopidogrel in Unstable Angina to Prevent Recurrent Events) trial, there was a 20% reduction in relative risk of death, non-fatal myocardial infarction and stroke with the addition of clopidogrel to aspirin. Some cardiologists advocate the use of 600 mg of clopidogrel for quicker and more effective antiplatelet effect. For those patients who are deemed at high risk on the basis of the TIMI score, additional antiplatelet inhibition can be achieved by using a glycoprotein IIb/IIIa receptor antagonist, such as tirofiban or eptifibatide prior to coronary angiography and coronary revascularization (so-called 'upstream treatment').

3. *Antithrombotic therapy.* Intravenous unfractionated heparin, with an activated partial thromboplastin time ratio of 1.5–2.5, results in a relative risk reduction of 70% in the incidence of myocardial infarction and refractory angina compared with placebo in patients with NSTEMI. However, low molecular weight heparins, such as subcutaneous enoxaparin (1 mg/kg BD), have more predictable bioavailability, obviating the need for monitoring (dose adjusted for body weight), are easier to administer and have been shown to be at least as effective as unfractionated heparin. Hence, low molecular weight heparin has largely replaced the use of unfractionated heparin for the treatment of acute coronary syndrome.

4. *Anti-anginal therapy.* Patients should receive β-blockers and nitrates, unless contraindicated. β-blockers blunt the sympathetic response and may reduce myocardial ischaemia by reducing heart rate, blood pressure and myocardial oxygen demand. β-blockers may also have anti-arrhythmic properties. An initial starting dose of metoprolol 25–50 mg BD should be uptitrated as tolerated. However, more unstable patients can either receive intravenous metoprolol (5–10 mg) or an intravenous infusion of esmolol at a rate of 50–200 µg/kg per minute. Coronary vasodilators are effective at relieving symptoms of chest pain but none of the following vasodilators have been shown to reduce myocardial infarction or improve survival.

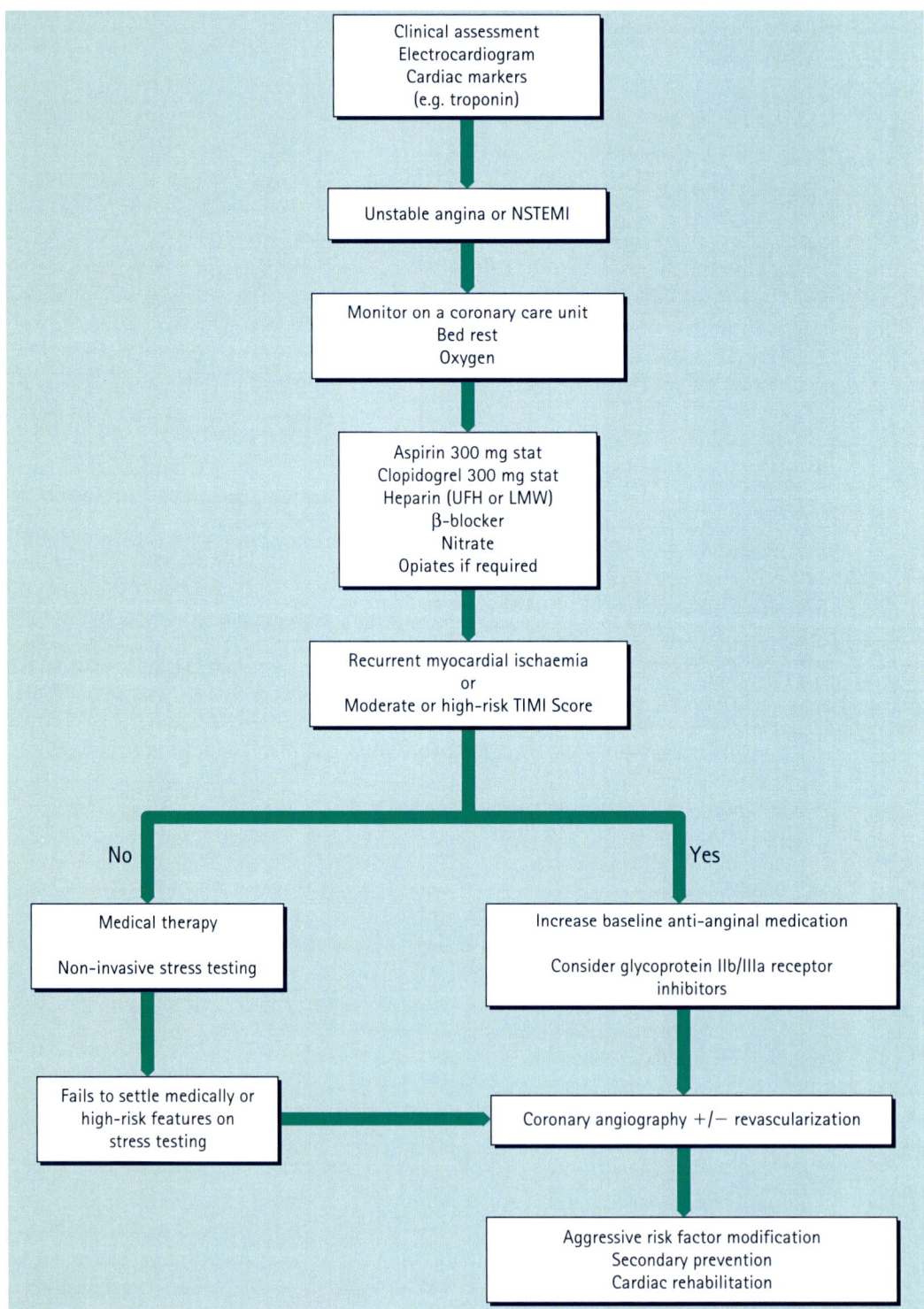

Figure 6.3 Summary of the treatment of patients with unstable angina and NSTEMI. LMW, low-molecular weight; NSTEMI, non-ST elevation myocardial infarction; TIMI (trial), Thrombolysis in Myocardial Infarction; UFH, unfractionated heparin.

- Nitrates should be the first-line vasodilator treatment with the mode of administration dictated by the patient's symptoms. Four to eight hundred micrograms of sublingual glyceryl trinitrate (GTN) usually provides rapid relief of symptoms. However, patients may require an intravenous infusion of GTN to relieve their symptoms, followed by a once-daily sustained release oral preparation, such as isosorbide mononitrate SR 30–120 mg OD.
- Rate-limiting calcium antagonists, such as diltiazem or verapamil, should be avoided in patients already on β-blockers due to the risk of serious bradycardia but may be useful in patients where β-blockers are contraindicated. Calcium channel antagonists, such as amlodipine 5–10 mg OD, may also reduce ischaemia.
- Potassium channel agonists (e.g. nicorandil 10–30 mg BD).

5 In patients with persistent chest pain unresponsive to nitrates and β-blockers, opiate analgesia with anti-emetics can be used (diamorphine 2.5–5 mg with metoclopromide 10 mg IV). These patients should be considered for urgent coronary angiography with a view to revascularization.

6 Patients who present with unstable angina or NSTEMI should be considered for inpatient coronary angiography with a view to revascularization. Although medical therapy may be considered first-line treatment in patients at low risk (from risk stratification), coronary angiography and revascularization should be offered to patients with persistent symptoms despite optimal medical therapy. Early coronary angiography should be undertaken in medium- to high-risk patients, as early coronary revascularization is associated with a reduction in the rate of subsequent myocardial infarction and death. Patients with single or two-vessel coronary artery disease with suitable coronary anatomy may be revascularized with percutaneous transluminal coronary angioplasty and stenting. However, patients with left main stem stenosis (50% stenosis or more), three-vessel coronary artery disease or two-vessel coronary artery disease, including the proximal left anterior descending artery, should be offered coronary artery bypass graft surgery, particularly in the context of impaired left ventricular systolic function and diabetes mellitus.

This patient was treated with aspirin, clopidogrel, enoxaparin and β-blockers. In view of persistent symptoms, she was commenced on intravenous nitrates and tirofiban. She subsequently underwent coronary angiography and uncomplicated coronary stenting to her left anterior descending artery.

Recent Developments

Antiplatelet therapy is central to the treatment of acute coronary syndromes. The benefit of clopidogrel, a thienopyridine in acute coronary syndrome has been confirmed in a number of clinical studies. More recently, prasugrel, which is a novel thienopyridine has been compared against clopidogrel in the TRITON TIMI-38 (TRial to assess Improvement in Therapeutic Outcomes by optimising platelet iNhibition with prasugrel – Thrombolysis In Myocardial Infarction 38) trial of 13 608 patients with acute coronary syndromes. Prasugrel was associated with significant reduction in the primary endpoint of cardiovascular death, myocardial infarction and stroke (9.9% versus 12.1%), largely due to the reduction in myocardial infarction. There was also a significant reduction in stent thrombosis with prasugrel. However, prasugrel was associated with significantly higher bleeding complications compared with clopidogrel, including life-threatening bleeds (1.4% versus 0.9%) and fatal bleeds (0.4% versus 0.1%). Hence, prasugrel may have a role in patients at high risk of recurrent ischaemic events, particularly if the risk of bleeding is low.

Conclusion

Patients presenting with symptoms suggestive of acute coronary syndrome should be risk-stratified, which will then guide subsequent therapy. Treatment should include antiplatelet, antithrombotic and anti-ischaemic agents. Early coronary angiography and revascularization should be considered in patients at high risk of infarction and death. Clinical symptoms with elevation in troponin are generally used to define myocardial infarction, but normal troponin measurement does not exclude an acute coronary syndrome.

Further Reading

Mehta SR, Cannon CP, Fox KA, *et al.* Routine vs selective invasive strategies in patients with acute coronary syndromes: a collaborative meta-analysis of randomized trials. *JAMA* 2005; **293**: 2908–17.

Qayyum R, Khalid MR, Adomaityte J, Papadakos SP, Messineo FC. Systematic review: comparing routine and selective invasive strategies for the acute coronary syndrome. *Ann Intern Med* 2008; **148**: 186–96.

PROBLEM

07 Initial management of ST elevation myocardial infarction

Case History

A 79-year-old woman presented with a 10-hour history of aching in her chest with heaviness in her arms associated with retching and sweating. She was overweight with a body mass index of 32 kg/m², had a history of hypertension and type 2 diabetes. Her regular medications include aspirin, simvastatin, ramipril and gliclazide. On examination, she looked slightly pale and sweaty, with a blood pressure of 110/78 mmHg and a heart

07 Initial management of ST elevation myocardial infarction

rate of 92 beats/minute. Her jugular venous pressure was not elevated and her chest was clear. Her electrocardiogram (ECG) is shown in Figure 7.1.

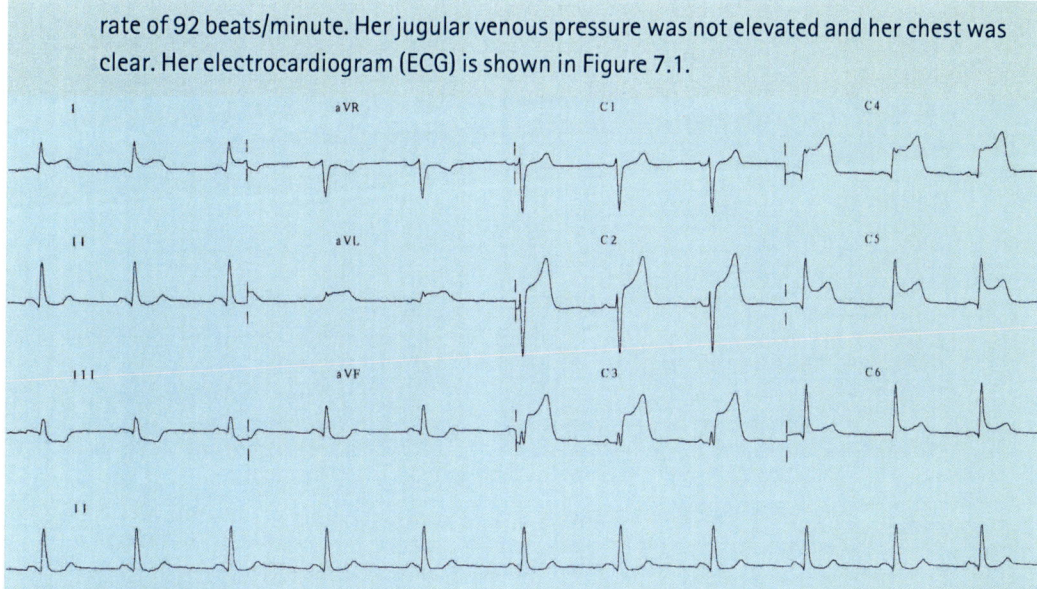

Figure 7.1 Anterior MI, ST segment elevation throughout precordial leads with reciprocal ST depression in the inferior leads (II, III and aVF).

What is the diagnosis?

What is the initial management for this patient?

What are the indications for reperfusion therapy?

What type of reperfusion treatment would you employ?

What are the absolute and relative contraindications to thrombolysis?

Sixty minutes following thrombolysis, the patient's ECG is unchanged with ongoing chest pain: What is the diagnosis?

What additional treatment has prognostic benefit?

How would you manage this patient's diabetes mellitus?

Background

 The clinical presentation and electrocardiographic changes are consistent with an acute anterolateral ST elevation myocardial infarction (STEMI). The paucity of symptoms is not unusual in the context of diabetes and advanced age.

What is the initial management for this patient?

Acute STEMI is a result of coronary artery occlusion and consequent myocardial necrosis (Figure 7.2). The complications of STEMI are related to the loss of myocardium, which may compromise pump function and provide the substrate for arrhythmias. The treatment of acute STEMI should be aimed at relieving coronary artery occlusion and treat-

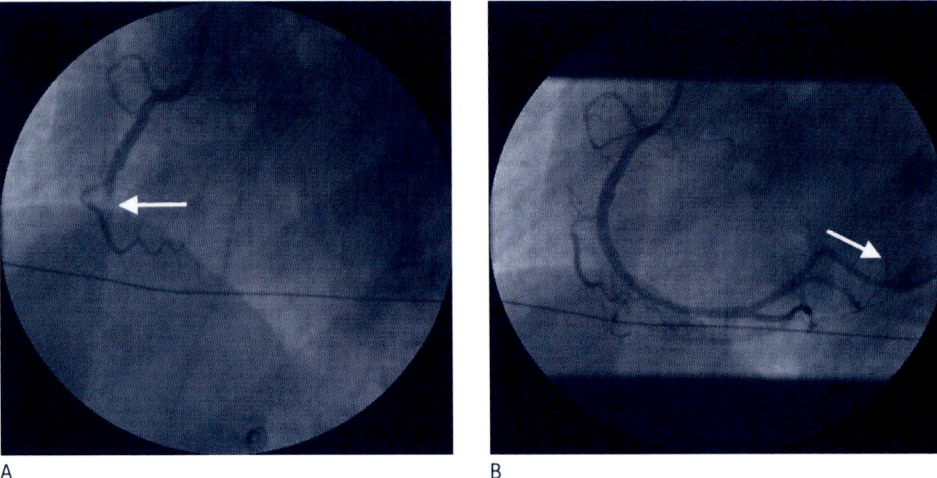

Figure 7.2 (A) Coronary angiogram demonstrating occlusion of the right coronary artery (arrow), which would typically result in ST elevation in leads II, III and aVF (inferior myocardial infarction). (B) Successful primary angioplasty with restoration of flow in the right coronary artery. Note the angioplasty wire *in situ* (arrow).

ment of complications (e.g. arrhythmias). Patients are at high risk of ventricular fibrillation or ventricular tachycardia within the first 24 hours after a STEMI and, therefore, patients should be monitored on a coronary care unit. Indeed, the development of coronary care units was prompted by the need for more rapid detection and treatment of ventricular arrhythmias, which led to significant improvements in survival from acute STEMI. Treatment should include supportive measures with oxygen therapy and analgesia (e.g. diamorphine 2.5–5 mg with the anti-emetic metoclopramide 10 mg) and specific anti-ischaemic, antiplatelet and reperfusion therapy.

A loading dose of aspirin 300 mg should be administered with 75 mg OD thereafter. In the ISIS-2 study (Second International Study of Infarct Survival), aspirin was shown to be almost as effective as streptokinase in reducing 30-day mortality following an acute STEMI. The benefit of aspirin and streptokinase combination was additive in this study. The COMMIT study (Clopidogrel and Metoprolol in Myocardial Infarction Trial) showed that the addition of clopidogrel (300 mg followed by 75 mg OD) to aspirin and thrombolysis further reduced cardiovascular morbidity and mortality. Hence, patients with acute myocardial infarction should also be treated with clopidogrel.

What are the indications for reperfusion therapy?

Reperfusion therapy should be considered when there is a typical history of ischaemic cardiac chest pain with the onset within 12 hours and an ECG showing one or more of the following:

1. 1-mm ST segment elevation in two or more adjacent limb leads (I, II, III, aVR, aVL and aVF).
2. 2-mm ST segment elevation in two or more adjacent chest leads (V1–6).
3. New-onset bundle branch block.
4. Dominant R waves and ST depression in V1–3 ('true posterior' MI).

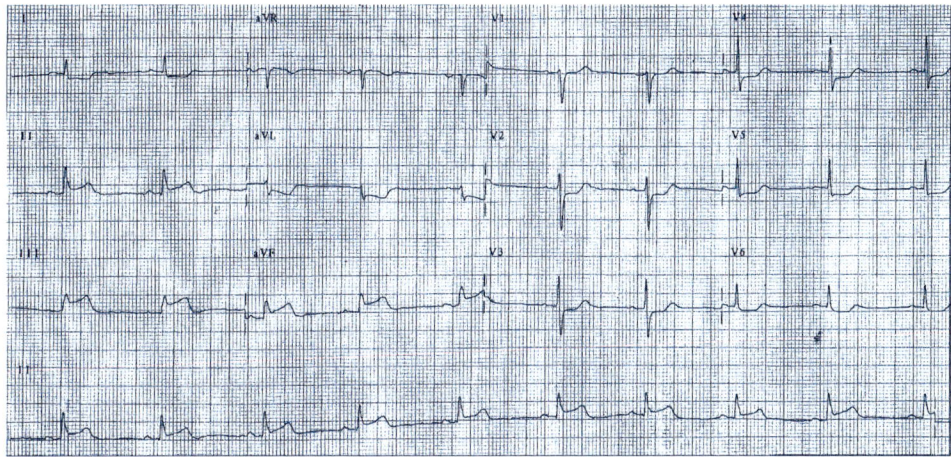

Figure 7.3 Inferior myocardial infarction, ST elevation in II, III and aVF with reciprocal depression in the precordial leads.

The degree of ST segment elevation and the number of leads involved is a surrogate marker for the amount of myocardium at risk. The above parameters would indicate sufficient risk of adverse outcome due to the MI to justify the risk associated with reperfusion therapy. Hence, this patient would be eligible for reperfusion therapy.

The electrocardiogram may be used for localization of the MI, which may indicate the occluded coronary artery. Anterior MI (usually left anterior descending artery territory) is indicated by ST segment elevation in the precordial leads, from V1 or V2 and may extend to V5 and V6 (Figure 7.1). There may be ST segment depression in the inferior leads. Inferior MI (right coronary artery or less commonly left circumflex coronary artery territory) typically involves ST elevation in leads II, III and aVF (Figure 7.3) and sometimes with reciprocal ST depression in V1 to V3.

What type of reperfusion treatment would you employ?

Primary percutaneous coronary intervention (PPCI) is now the chosen first-line therapy for STEMI. In comparison with thrombolysis, PPCI is associated with lower rates of re-infarction, stroke, major bleeding and death. Ideally, patients with a STEMI should be transferred directly to a centre equipped to perform PPCI. However, inter-hospital transfers introduce delays to treatment that may compromise clinical outcomes. Studies suggest that inter-hospital transfer may be undertaken if balloon inflation within the occluded coronary vessel can be achieved within 120 minutes of the patient symptoms. Thrombolysis should be considered if significant delays are anticipated. For optimal outcomes, a PPCI service should offer a first door to balloon time of less than 90 minutes. PPCI is often performed with adjunctive heparin and glycoprotein IIb/IIIa antagonist (abciximab) therapy. Hence, the risk of bleeding, although lower than that of thrombolysis, remains significant.

With thrombolysis, an accelerated regimen of tissue plasminogen activator administered over 90 minutes, or a single bolus of weight-adjusted tenecteplase, are the thrombolytic agents of choice for acute STEMI (Figure 7.4). These should be administered with a bolus followed by an infusion of intravenous unfractionated heparin. Thrombolysis

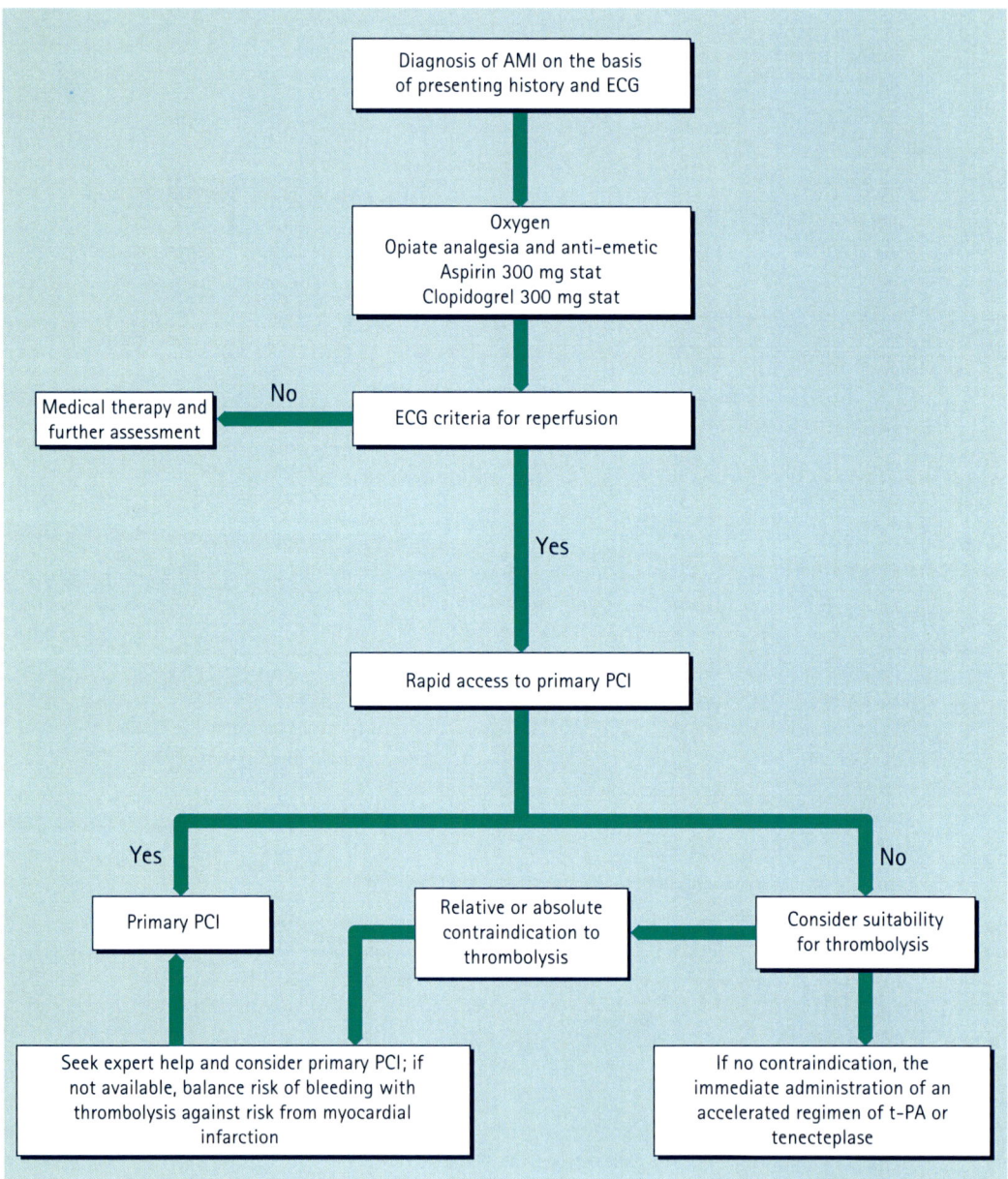

Figure 7.4 Algorithm for the management of STEMI. AMI, acute myocardial infarction; PCI, percutaneous coronary intervention; t-PA, tissue plasminogen activator.

should be administered at the earliest opportunity once the diagnosis has been confirmed. The benefit of thrombolysis is time dependent, with the greatest benefit in patients who receive treatment within 3 hours of the onset of chest pain. The current standard for in-hospital thrombolysis is for the patient to have thrombolysis administered within 20 minutes of arrival at hospital (door to needle time). Benefit, in terms of mortality reduction, reduces rapidly over the next 3–12 hours following the onset of chest pain. Thrombolysis should only be considered in patients who present 12–24 hours following the onset of chest pain if there is ongoing chest pain with evolving ST segment elevation. The time-dependent benefit of thrombolysis has led to the development of pre-hospital thrombolysis administered by paramedic crews, particularly in more remote areas of the country, where transfer times to hospital are long.

What are the absolute and relative contraindications to thrombolysis?

Absolute contraindications are as follows:

- Active internal bleeding or gastrointestinal bleeding within the last month.
- Haemorrhagic stroke at any time in the past or ischaemic stroke within the last 6 months.
- Bleeding diathesis.
- Major surgery, including abdominal, neurological or eye surgery, in the last month.
- Known or suspected aortic dissection.
- Acute pancreatitis or severe liver disease.
- Intracranial neoplasm.

Relative contraindications are as follows:

- Severe hypertension (systolic blood pressure >200 mmHg or diastolic blood pressure >100 mmHg). Intravenous β-blockers or intravenous nitrates should be used to reduce blood pressure and, once controlled, thrombolysis should be administered.
- Trauma (e.g. from prolonged cardiopulmonary resuscitation >10 min).
- Known abdominal aortic aneurysm.
- Advanced liver disease.

Concurrent anticoagulant therapy, pregnancy and proliferative diabetic retinopathy are not absolute contraindications to thrombolysis.

For patients who have a relative contraindication to thrombolysis, the balance of bleeding risk should be weighed against the risk associated with the MI. For patients with an absolute or relative contraindication to thrombolysis, a specialist opinion should be sought to decide on the appropriateness of primary angioplasty.

Sixty minutes following thrombolysis, the patient's ECG is unchanged with ongoing chest pain: What is the diagnosis?

Resolution of ST segment elevation is related to restoration of myocardial blood flow and perfusion. Generally, a threshold of 50% reduction in maximum ST segment elevation or resolution of the acute bundle branch block has been used as a surrogate measure of successful reperfusion therapy. If this fails to occur, particularly if the patient has ongoing chest pain, then the patient is deemed to have failed reperfusion. Based on the results of the REACT trial (Rescue Angioplasty Versus Conservative Treatment or Repeat Thrombolysis), patients with failed thrombolytic therapy should be referred for emergency coronary intervention. Coronary intervention following failed reperfusion therapy with thrombolysis is termed 'rescue angioplasty'. While awaiting rescue angioplasty, aggressive medical management may be required. Approximately one-third of patients treated with thrombolysis will fail to demonstrate reperfusion (by the ECG criteria) and thus require rescue angioplasty.

Table 7.1 Killip classification of patients with acute myocardial infarction

Class	Definition
I	Triple rhythm with absent rales
II	Rales over less than 50% of the lung fields
III	Rales over more than 50% of the lung fields
IV	Shock

What additional treatment has prognostic benefit?

β-blockers

A meta-analysis of randomized controlled trials, involving in excess of 52 000 patients, showed early β-blocker treatment given to patients with STEMI in Killip Class I (Table 7.1) with a heart rate >65 beats/minute and blood pressure >105 mmHg, initially intravenously and then orally, reduced mortality by 70%. There was a similar reduction in ventricular arrhythmias, cardiac arrests and a reduction in reinfarction of 50%. However, the recent COMMIT study failed to confirm the benefit of metoprolol (intravenous followed by oral metoprolol) of this magnitude in patients with STEMI. This study showed reduction in reinfarction and ventricular arrhythmias but significant increase in cardiogenic shock, particularly in patients with signs of heart failure. Hence, acute (within 24 hours) β-blocker treatment should be considered only in the absence of heart failure, hypotension or bradyarrhythmia.

Angiotension-converting enzyme inhibitors

Angiotension-converting enzyme inhibitors improve long-term prognosis in patients following a MI. Although not restricted to patients with impaired left ventricular systolic function, the benefit appears to be greatest in this group of patients. In the absence of significant hypotension, angiotension-converting enzyme inhibitors should be initiated in the first 36 hours of admission (e.g. ramipril 1.25 mg uptitrating to 5 mg BD as tolerated), particularly in patients with heart failure and left ventricular dysfunction.

In patients intolerant to angiotension-converting enzyme inhibitor therapy, an angiotensin II receptor antagonist should be used. Valsartan has been shown to be an effective alternative to an angiotension-converting enzyme inhibitor in patients with MI and left ventricular dysfunction.

Aldosterone receptor antagonist

Eplerenone 25 mg OD, uptitrated to 50 mg OD, should be commenced within 3–14 days of a STEMI, and continued for 16 months, in all patients with an echocardiogram ejection fraction of <40% and clinical evidence of heart failure or diabetes mellitus. This results in a significant reduction in all-cause mortality and hospitalization (EPHESUS [Eplerenone Post-Acute Myocardial Infarction Heart Failure Efficacy and Survival Study]).

How would you manage this patient's diabetes mellitus?

On admission, elevated blood glucose is associated with a significant increase in risk of mortality. Although the benefit of aggressive blood glucose control has not been conclusively demonstrated, 24 hours of insulin infusion for glycaemic control is generally rec-

Table 7.2 Recommended regimen for insulin intravenous infusion	
Blood glucose (mmol/l)	Infusion rate (units/hour)
<4	0.5
4.1–8	1
8.1–12	2
12.1–16	3
16.1–20	4
20.1–24	6
>24	8

ommended for patients with diabetes or presentation blood glucose of 11 mmol/l or more. Thereafter, either insulin or oral hypoglycaemics may be introduced and up-titrated to achieve control of blood glucose. For the first 24 hours, an intravenous infusion of actrapid 50 units in 50 ml of normal saline (with the rate being titrated with blood glucose) should be administered. Blood glucose should be checked every 2 hours with the dose of insulin adjusted accordingly. An example of intravenous insulin infusion rates is provided in Table 7.2. Of note, metformin should be avoided or withheld for 48 hours in patients undergoing coronary angiography and angioplasty due to the risk of lactic acidosis when used in conjunction with intravenous contrast.

Recent Developments

PPCI for acute STEMI is generally regarded as the 'gold standard' treatment. However, it is not as widely available as thrombolysis. A strategy of transferring patients to a centre for PPCI was compared against on-site thrombolysis in the DANAMI-2 study (Danish Trial in Acute Myocardial Infarction-2). This study showed that transfer to a centre for PPCI was safe and more effective than on-site thrombolysis if the transfer can be accomplished in less than 2 hours. More recently, a registry study from France suggests that a strategy of early thrombolysis followed by coronary angiography and PCI (generally within 24 hours) may produce clinical outcomes comparable with PPCI. Hence, initial thrombolysis may be as effective as PPCI if coupled with transfer to a centre for angiography and PCI.

Pharmacological facilitation of PCI (i.e. administration of thrombolytic and/or glycoprotein IIb/IIIa inhibitors prior to PCI) has also been studied. The FINESSE study (Facilitated Intervention with Enhanced Reperfusion Speed to Stop Events) randomized 2452 patients with STEMI to facilitation with reteplase–abciximab or abciximab alone, or PPCI without facilitation. There was no significant difference in clinical outcome.

Conclusion

Acute STEMI should be managed as a medical emergency and treatment should include a combination of general supportive measures (e.g. oxygen and analgesia), anti-ischaemic, antiplatelet and reperfusion therapy. Patients are at risk of arrhythmias and pump failure following STEMI and should be closely monitored. PPCI is widely regarded as the most effective strategy for reperfusion, and rescue angioplasty should be offered if thrombolysis is utilized as the primary mode of reperfusion therapy. Minimizing the time to treatment is crucial regardless of the reperfusion therapy.

Further Reading

Antman EM, Hand M, Armstrong PW, *et al*; 2004 Writing Committee Members, Anbe DT, Kushner FG, Ornato JP, *et al.* 2007 focused Update of the ACC/AHA 2004 Guidelines for the Management of Patients With ST-Elevation Myocardial Infarction: a report of the American College of Cardiology/American Heart Association Task Force on Practice Guidelines: developed in collaboration with the Canadian Cardiovascular Society endorsed by the American Academy of Family Physicians: 2007 Writing Group to Review New Evidence and Update the ACC/AHA 2004 Guidelines for the Management of Patients With ST-Elevation Myocardial Infarction, Writing on Behalf of the 2004 Writing Committee. *Circulation* 2008; **117**: 296–329.

PROBLEM

08 Hypotension in acute myocardial infarction

Case History

A 58-year-old man presented with a 6-hour history of central chest pain. His electrocardiogram (ECG) showed an acute inferior ST elevation myocardial infarction with the development of early Q waves. He underwent immediate coronary angiography, which showed a moderate stenosis in the left anterior descending artery with an occluded proximal right coronary artery. The patient then underwent primary angioplasty and stent deployment to the proximal right coronary artery. On return to the ward, his blood pressure was noted to be low at 84/50 mmHg, with a pulse of 100 beats/minute. His jugular venous pressure was elevated and his chest was clear.

What is the cause of his hypotension?

How would you manage this patient?

Background

In any patient who has undergone coronary intervention and then develops hypotension, the possibility of a bleeding complication or cardiac tamponade should be considered and excluded. Causes and diagnosis of hypotension are listed in Table 8.1.

Bleeding complications from arterial access for coronary intervention should always be considered, particularly if the femoral artery was used as the access site. The use of heparins and multiple antiplatelet agents significantly increases the risk of bleeding. Significant blood loss into the retroperitoneal space can occur without overt external bleeding. Radial artery access for coronary intervention is associated with a lower risk of bleeding complications.

The most likely diagnosis is that of a right ventricular infarct resulting from extensive damage to the right ventricle, usually caused by a proximal occlusion of the right coronary artery, as in this case. With impaired right ventricular systolic function, there is reduced left ventricular filling pressure resulting in systemic hypotension, with an elevated jugular venous pressure and hepatic congestion without evidence of pulmonary congestion.

This can be confirmed on an ECG with right-sided chest leads (V4R–V6R), which may show residual ST segment elevation with Q waves. Echocardiography shows a dilated right ventricle with reduced systolic function and is usually associated with tricuspid regurgitation. The left ventricle may also be impaired and the absence of pulmonary

Table 8.1 Causes of hypotension in acute myocardial infarction

Cause	Diagnostic modality
Cardiogenic shock due to: 1 Extensive left ventricular myocardial infarction 2 Right ventricular infarction 3 Ventricular septal rupture 4 Free wall rupture 5 Acute severe mitral regurgitation	Clinical examination, ECG, echocardiography, right heart catheterization
Spontaneous haemorrhage due to antiplatelet, antithrombotic and thrombolytic therapy 1 Retroperitoneal 2 Gastrointestinal	Clinical history and examination; ultrasound or CT for retroperitoneal haemorrhage
Aortic dissection causing tamponade/rupture (rarely aortic dissection may present as acute myocardial infarction due to dissection of coronary ostia)	Echocardiography, CT
Massive pulmonary embolus	Clinical, echocardiography, CT pulmonary angiography
Complication of coronary angiography/angioplasty 1 Acute coronary artery occlusion 2 Vessel perforation and tamponade 3 Contrast media reaction 4 Vasovagal syncope after peripheral arterial cannulation 5 Haemorrhage at peripheral arterial access site	ECG, coronary angiography, echocardiography Most cases of contrast reaction are accompanied by a rash and other evidence of anaphylaxis
Tamponade due to right ventricular perforation by temporary pacemaker or central line	Echocardiography

CT, computed tomography.

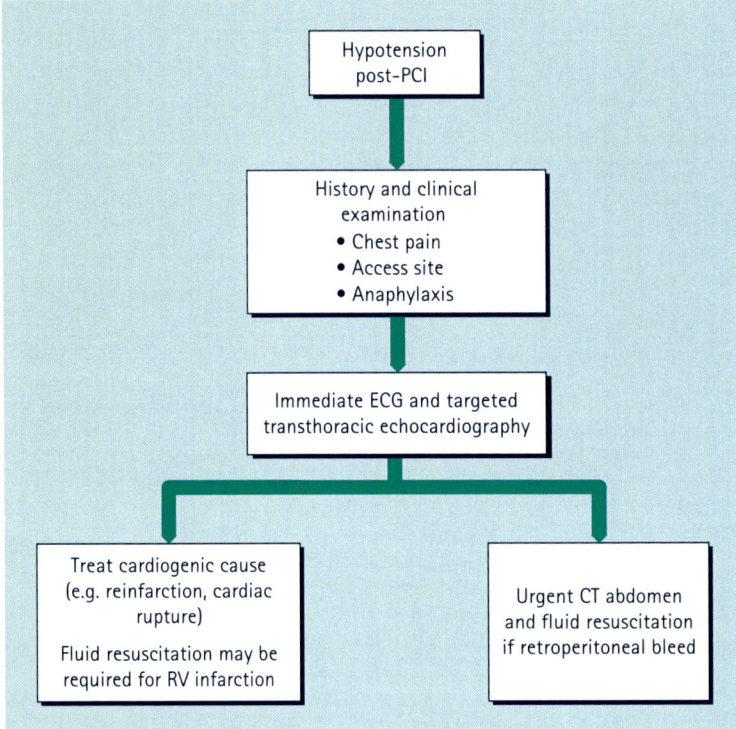

Figure 8.1 Management of hypotension post-myocardial infarction. CT, computed tomography; PCI, percutaneous coronary intervention; RV, right ventricular.

oedema, clinically or radiologically, does not necessarily imply normal left ventricular systolic function. Echocardiography is also useful to confirm or exclude other mechanical complications of myocardial infarction such as an acute ventricular septal defect or acute severe mitral regurgitation secondary to chordal or papillary muscle rupture.

How would you manage this patient?

If there is no evidence of pulmonary oedema, either clinically or radiologically, the treatment of choice is to increase left ventricular filling pressure with intravenous fluids using the right ventricle as a conduit to adequately fill the left ventricle. This can be achieved by administering aliquots of intravenous fluid, 100 ml at a time. More than a litre may be required to achieve adequate left ventricular filling pressures. If hypotension persists or pulmonary oedema occurs, then invasive pulmonary artery pressure monitoring with a pulmonary artery catheter should be utilized (Figure 8.1). If the pulmonary wedge pressure is <15 mmHg, then additional fluid may be administered, but higher pulmonary wedge pressures in the context of pulmonary oedema would suggest concomitant left ventricular impairment and inotropic support with an intra-aortic balloon pump should be considered.

Heart block and bradyarrhythmias are frequently observed in patients with inferior myocardial infarction and generally not well tolerated if there is concomitant right ventricular infarction. Temporary pacing should be considered in these patients.

Recent Developments

Bleeding is a major complication following coronary intervention (in the context of anti-platelet and anti-thrombotic therapy) and is associated with worse clinical outcomes. A transradial approach to coronary angiography and coronary intervention is associated with lower rates of major bleeding and vascular complications compared to transfemoral approach. Recent studies suggest that a transradial approach is safe even in the setting of acute myocardial infarction and primary percutaneous coronary intervention.

Conclusion

Hypotension in the setting of acute myocardial infarction has numerous causes and may not be cardiogenic in aetiology. Treatment should target the cause of hypotension. Right ventricular infarction should be considered, particularly in inferior myocardial infarction, as the right coronary artery, which supplies the right ventricle in the majority of cases, is often the culprit.

Further Reading

Andersen JL, Adams CD, Antman EM, *et al.* ACC/AHA 2007 guidelines for the management of patients with unstable angina/non-ST-elevation myocardial infarction: a report of the American College of Cardiology/American Heart Association Task Force on Practice Guidelines (Writing Committee to Revise the 2002 Guidelines for the Management of Patients With Unstable Angina/Non-ST-Elevation Myocardial Infarction) developed in collaboration with the American College of Emergency Physicians, the Society for Cardiovascular Angiography and Interventions, and the Society of Thoracic Surgeons endorsed by the American Association of Cardiovascular and Pulmonary Rehabilitation and the Society for Academic Emergency Medicine. *J Am Coll Cardiol* 2007; **50**: e1–157.

Jolly SS, Amlani S, Hamon M, Yusuf S, Mehta SR. Radial versus femoral access for coronary angiography or intervention and the impact on major bleeding and ischemic events: a systematic review and meta-analysis of randomised trials. *Am Heart J* 2009; **157**: 132–40.

PROBLEM

09 Cardiogenic shock

Case History

A 71-year-old man presented after 9 hours of chest pain and was diagnosed with an acute anterior ST elevation myocardial infarction. He has a history of hypercholesterolaemia and hypertension, treated normally with simvastatin and amlodipine. He was thrombolysed within 30 minutes of hospital admission with a weight-adjusted dose of tenecteplase, with heparin, resulting in 30% resolution in ST segment elevation. However, his clinical state deteriorated and he required 6 litres of oxygen to maintain oxygen saturations of >90%. His blood pressure deteriorated to 86/50 mmHg (from 110/76 mmHg on admission) and he became tachycardic with a heart rate of 126 beats/minute. His electrocardiogram (ECG) confirmed sinus tachycardia. He had crepitations to the mid zones of his chest and a gallop rhythm. There were no murmurs. His peripheries were cold and he was oliguric (urine output was 20 ml in the last hour).

How would you define his current clinical state?

What are the commonest causes of cardiogenic shock and their associated mortality?

How would you manage this patient?

Background

This patient has cardiogenic shock with a Killip classification of IV. Haemodynamically, cardiogenic shock may be defined by low cardiac output despite adequate ventricular filling, i.e. a low cardiac index (<2.2 l/min per m^2) and elevated pulmonary capillary wedge pressure, a surrogate of left atrial pressure (>15 mmHg). Clinically, cardiogenic shock can be identified by relative arterial hypotension (systolic blood pressure typically <90 mmHg), evidence of tissue hypoperfusion (e.g. cold, clammy peripheries and oliguria or anuria) and pulmonary congestion, although some patients with cardiogenic shock do not exhibit all these features. Of note, although the systolic blood pressure is usually <90 mm/Hg, clinical manifestations of tissue hypoperfusion may be more relevant than the actual systolic blood pressure.

Cardiogenic shock associated with a myocardial infarction is associated with a high mortality rate, even with aggressive treatment (30-day mortality of almost 50%). Many patients have three-vessel coronary artery disease, or left main stem disease. Although larger infarcts are more likely to precipitate cardiogenic shock, the diagnosis cannot be excluded based on infarct size alone. Cardiogenic shock is more common in those with a previous history of heart failure and in elderly patients.

What are the commonest causes of cardiogenic shock and their associated mortality?

Causes of cardiogenic shock are listed in Table 9.1 with their associated mortality (SHOCK [SHould we emergently revascularize Occluded Coronaries for shocK]) trial. The development of an acute ventricular septal defect with cardiogenic shock is associated with the worst outcome.

Table 9.1 Causes of cardiogenic shock

Cause of cardiogenic shock	% cases	Mortality (%)
Left ventricle failure	78.5	59.2
Acute severe mitral regurgitation	6.9	55.1
Ventricular septal defect	3.9	87.3
Right ventricle failure	2.8	55
Cardiac tamponade	1.4	55
Others	6.5	65.3

How would you manage this patient?

The haemodynamic compromise associated with cardiogenic shock results in tissue hypoperfusion resulting in acute tubular necrosis with deterioration in renal function and oliguria/anuria, extension of the myocardial infarction, acute ischaemic hepatic impairment and activation of systemic inflammatory response. Hence, cardiogenic shock is a systemic illness as a consequence of acute reduction in cardiac output.

Therefore, the haemodynamic status should be normalized as a matter of urgency to maintain tissue perfusion and oxygenation. The cause of cardiogenic shock should be identified and treated, which will require prompt echocardiographic examination. Acute ventricular septal defects, acute severe mitral regurgitation due to chordal or papillary muscle rupture, or free wall ruptures are cardiothoracic surgical emergencies. Any cardiac rhythm disturbance should be corrected in order to optimize cardiac function. This patient's echocardiogram confirmed severe left ventricle systolic impairment (Figure 9.1).

Oxygenation

All patients should receive high flow oxygen in order to achieve adequate oxygenation. Continuous pulse oximetry should be utilized, but this may not reflect central oxygenation due to poor peripheral perfusion and, therefore, arterial blood gases or an arterial line should be considered (beware of bleeding risk following thrombolysis). Caution should be exercised in patients who have chronic obstructive pulmonary disease with carbon dioxide retention. If despite high flow oxygen therapy the patient fails to achieve adequate oxygenation, then non-invasive continuous positive airways pressure ventilation should be considered. If the patient continues to become hypoxic with an increase in PCO_2, or worsening acidosis, then intubation and intermittent positive pressure ventilation with positive end-expiratory pressure should be utilized to clear alveoli oedema. This will improve oxygenation, reduce hypercapnia and restore pH balance.

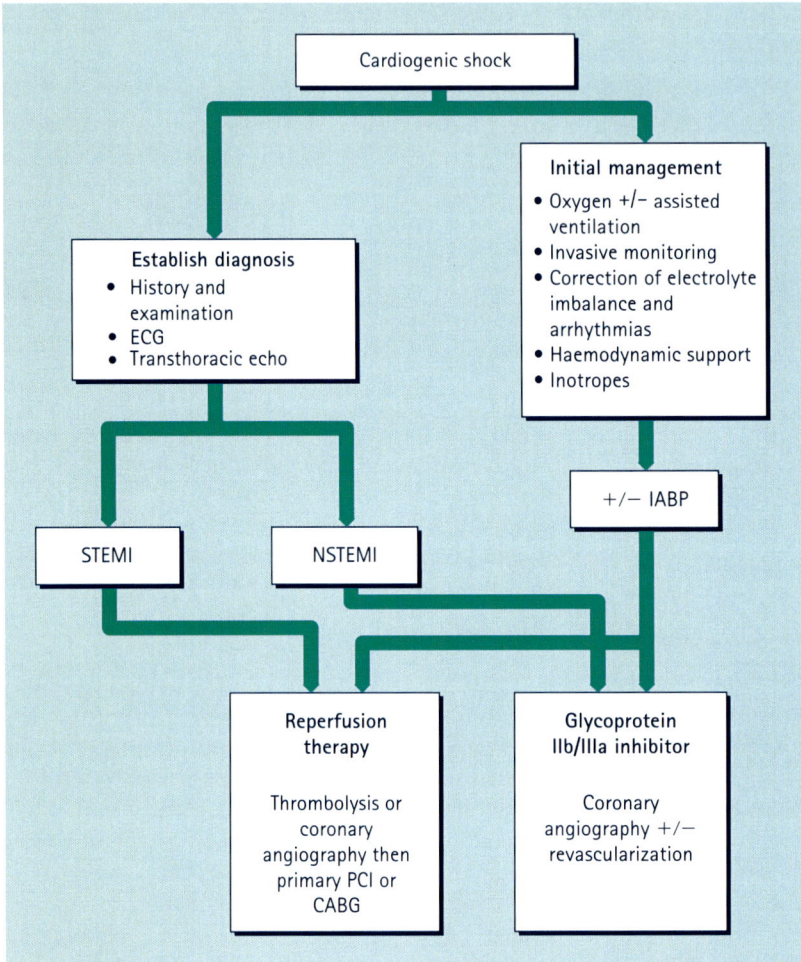

Figure 9.1 Algorithm for the management of cardiogenic shock. CABG, coronary artery bypass graft surgery; IABP, intra-aortic balloon pump; NSTEMI, non-ST elevation myocardial infarction; PCI, percutaneous coronary intervention; STEMI, ST elevation myocardial infarction.

Invasive monitoring (pulmonary artery catheterization)

Pulmonary artery catheters should be reserved for the management of selected patients with cardiogenic shock. Routine use of pulmonary artery catheters has not been shown to improve clinical outcomes and may even increase the risk of complications. The diagnosis of cardiogenic shock may be confirmed by the demonstration of low cardiac output (using thermodilution) and elevated left ventricular filling pressure (assessed by measuring pulmonary capillary wedge pressure). Of note, there are limitations to the use of pulmonary capillary wedge pressure to approximate left ventricular filling pressures and it should not be routinely used to guide fluid management in cardiogenic shock. Table 9.2 details the interpretation of right heart catheter data. A cardiac index of <2.2 l/min per m^2 and an elevated wedge pressure of >25 mmHg are associated with poor prognosis.

Table 9.2 Interpretation of right heart data obtained with a pulmonary artery catheter

	CVP	PCWP	CO	SVR	A-V SaO$_2$
Left ventricle failure	↑	↑	↓	↑	↑
Right ventricle failure	↑	↓	↓	↑	↑
Cardiac tamponade	↑	↑	↓	↑	↑
Acquired VSD	↑	↑	↓	↑	↓
Hypovolaemia	↓	↓	↓	↑	↑
Septicaemia	↓	↓	↑	↓	↓

A-V SaO$_2$, difference between arterial and mixed venous oxygen saturations; CO, cardiac output; CVP, central venous pressure; SVR, systemic vascular resistance; VSD, ventricular septal defect.

Inotropic support

If, despite adequate filling of the left ventricle, the systemic blood pressure remains low with evidence of tissue hypoperfusion, inotropic therapy (dobutamine 2.5–20 µg/kg per minute) should be considered. Dobutamine, a β-adrenergic agonist, increases the force of cardiac contraction with peripheral vasodilatation, thus reducing afterload. The addition of dopamine (1–3 µg/kg per minute) improves renal blood flow and is positively inotropic, but peripheral vasoconstriction at higher doses may be detrimental as it increases afterload. Administration of dopamine must only be through a central venous catheter as extravasation from a peripheral vein causes severe tissue necrosis.

Phosphodiesterase inhibitors (e.g. milrinone) offer an alternative to dobutamine, particularly in patients treated with β-blockers. They are positively inotropic in addition to being vasodilatory. Of note, inotropic agents may improve haemodynamics but increase oxygen consumption and may exacerbate myocardial ischaemia. These agents may also precipitate arrhythmias.

Intra-aortic balloon pump counterpulsation

An intra-aortic balloon pump (IABP) consists of a large balloon (34, 40 or 50 ml, depending on the patient's height), which is introduced via the femoral artery into the descending thoracic aorta (Figure 9.2). This balloon inflates with helium during diastole and deflates in systole, which results in counterpulsation. Balloon inflation during diastole augments diastolic blood pressure and increases blood flow, and balloon deflation in systole reduces afterload. As coronary blood flow occurs predominantly in diastole, coronary blood flow and perfusion may be improved by IABP. Balloon inflation can be triggered by the aortic pressure waveform or by the ECG.

Contraindications to IABP include severe peripheral vascular disease, aortic dissection or aneurysm and severe aortic regurgitation, as the latter is worsened by diastolic counterpulsation. Complications relate to the risk of infection, haemorrhage at the vascular access site, peripheral vascular complications such as distal limb ischaemia and aortic dissection or perforation. The current guidelines recommend early IABP insertion as a class 1 indication for patients in cardiogenic shock.

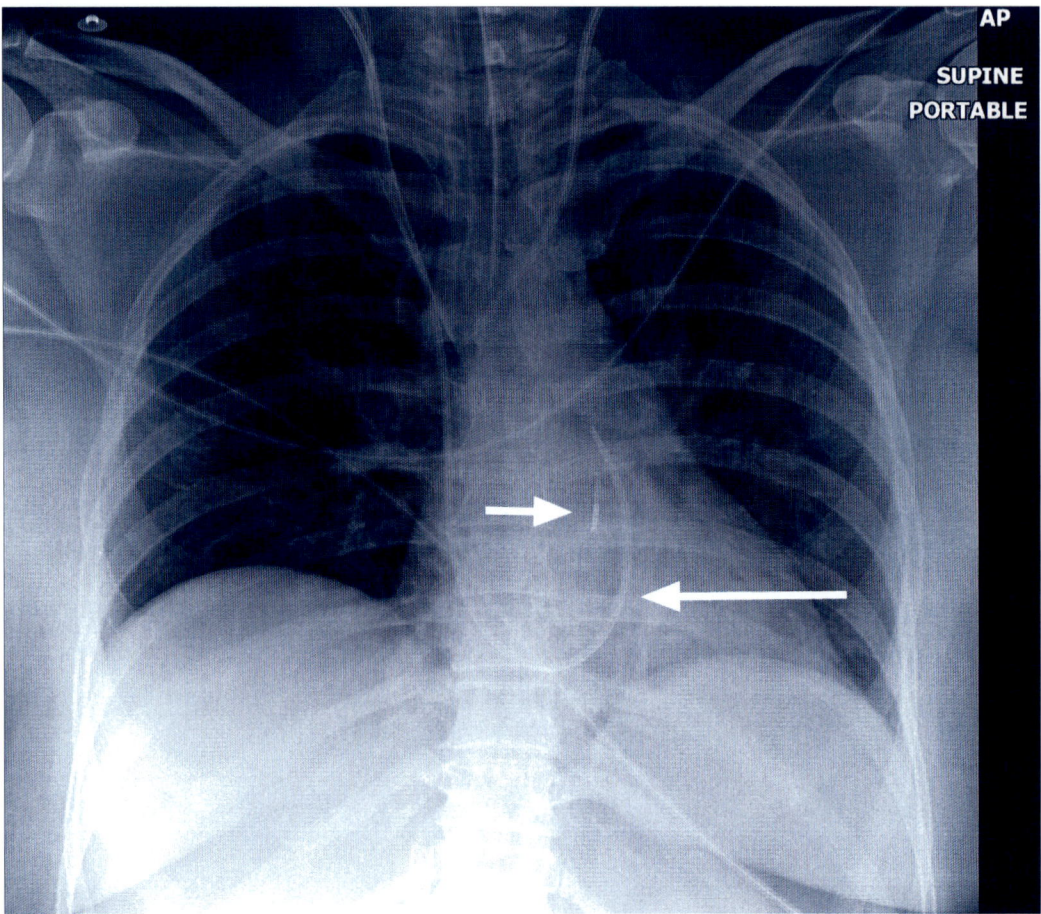

Figure 9.2 Radio-opaque marker of the intra-aortic balloon pump in the descending aorta (short arrow). A pulmonary artery catheter (Swan–Ganz catheter) is in the pulmonary artery (long arrow) via the right internal jugular vein.

Renal support

If patients fail to achieve an adequate urine output despite optimization of haemodynamic status, and continue to have pulmonary oedema, then this can be managed by haemofiltration with a negative fluid balance.

Revascularization

The SHOCK trial compared 'medical stabilization' against 'emergency revascularization' in patients with cardiogenic shock within 36 hours of myocardial infarction. In this study, 'emergency revascularization' was associated with lower mortality rates compared with medical therapy. By 12 months, there was a significant survival benefit with early revascularization (47% versus 34%; $P = 0.025$) with 132 lives saved per 1000 patients. Hence, all patients with cardiogenic shock should be considered for revascularization. Of note, IABP was used in >85% of cases and >37% of patients were revascularized by coronary artery bypass graft surgery.

Recent Developments

Cardiogenic shock is associated with a systemic inflammatory response with increased expression of inducible nitric oxide synthase and generation of excess nitric oxide, which may contribute to the pathogenesis of cardiogenic shock. This has prompted investigations into nitric oxide synthase inhibitors (e.g. tilarginine), but clinical studies have failed to demonstrate survival benefit with these agents.

There is also increasing interest in percutaneous left ventricular assist devices, which may provide greater haemodynamic support than IABPs. However, these devices are more complex and associated with a greater risk of vascular complications.

Conclusion

Cardiogenic shock is a medical emergency. This clinical syndrome should be recognized early and treated promptly. Urgent haemodynamic support, including inotropic agents and IABP, should be coupled with urgent revascularization. The latter has been shown to improve survival. However, despite aggressive medical therapy, mortality rates remain unacceptably high.

Further Reading

Antman EM, Hand M, Armstrong PW, *et al*; 2004 Writing Committee Members, Anbe DT, Kushner FG, Ornato JP, *et al.* 2007 focused Update of the ACC/AHA 2004 Guidelines for the Management of Patients With ST-Elevation Myocardial Infarction: a report of the American College of Cardiology/American Heart Association Task Force on Practice Guidelines: developed in collaboration with the Canadian Cardiovascular Society endorsed by the American Academy of Family Physicians: 2007 Writing Group to Review New Evidence and Update the ACC/AHA 2004 Guidelines for the Management of Patients With ST-Elevation Myocardial Infarction, Writing on Behalf of the 2004 Writing Committee. *Circulation* 2008; **117**: 296–329.

Hochman JS, Sleeper LA, Webb JG, *et al*. Early revascularization in acute myocardial infarction complicated by cardiogenic shock. *N Engl J Med* 1999; **341**: 625–34.

10 Peri-infarct arrhythmia

Case History

A 56-year-old man, who had been thrombolysed for an inferior ST elevation myocardial infarction 2 hours earlier, was noted to be bradycardic with a heart rate of about 50 beats/minute. He had more than 50% reduction of his ST segment elevation and almost complete resolution of chest pain. His blood pressure was stable at 110/72 mmHg and he was not symptomatic of his bradycardia. A rhythm strip was acquired and is shown in Figure 10.1.

How would you manage this patient?

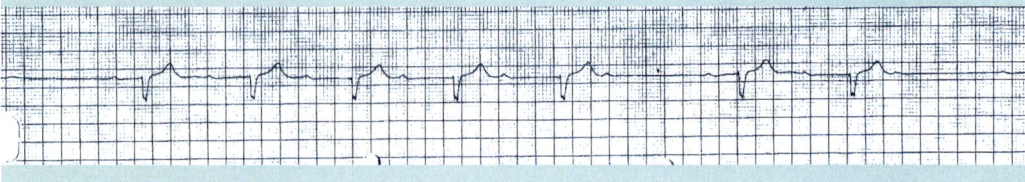

Figure 10.1 Wenckebach conduction.

Closer inspection will reveal (subtle) prolongation of the PR interval preceding the non-conducted P waves. Hence, this patient has developed second-degree heart block with Wenckebach conduction.

Background

Atrioventricular conduction abnormalities are not uncommon during acute myocardial infarction, particularly in association with inferior myocardial infarctions. The rhythm strip shows a long PR interval and intermittent non-conducted P waves. In general, atrioventricular conduction abnormalities in the context of an inferior ST segment elevation myocardial infarction do not necessarily imply larger infarction and seldom require treatment, as they are generally well tolerated and tend to resolve with reperfusion therapy. Resolution of conduction abnormality tends to occur in a stepwise fashion sometimes over 7–10 days, i.e. from complete heart block to Mobitz II and Mobitz I block, then first-degree heart block and normal conduction. Permanent pacing is unusual in inferior myocardial infarction and reserved for patients who fail to improve after this period of time. However, in rare cases of heart block with evidence of haemodynamic compromise in inferior myocardial infarction, intravenous atropine and even a temporary pacing wire may be required. Aminophylline has also been used with some success as the antagonism of endogenous adenosine (released during infarction) may improve atrioventricular conduction in inferior myocardial infarction, but should not be regarded as first-line treatment in a patient with haemodynamic compromise. β-blocker therapy should be withheld if there is evidence of conduction abnormality.

In contrast, complete heart block in the context of a recent anterior myocardial infarction is usually the result of more extensive myocardial infarction and direct damage to the conduction tissue. Complete heart block in patients with anterior myocardial infarction is often associated with a slower and broader QRS escape rhythm, which is more likely to be associated with haemodynamic compromise (probably due to a combination of compromised pump function from extensive myocardial damage and bradyarrhythmia) and progression to asystole. Hence, temporary pacing is usually required. Response to intravenous atropine is usually limited. The risk of progression to complete heart block and asystole is also high following an anterior ST elevation myocardial infarction in the context of new bifascicular block (right bundle branch block with left or right axis deviation) and trifascicular block (e.g. alternating bundle branch block). Therefore, temporary pacing should be considered in these patients. As conduction abnormalities are a result of conduction tissue damage (and unlikely to improve), these patients will usually require permanent pacemaker implantation.

Other arrhythmias are common in the setting of acute myocardial infarction. β-blockers may reduce ventricular arrhythmias and should be used in the absence of contraindications. Ventricular extrasystoles and tachycardia (particularly non-sustained ventricular tachycardia, i.e. <30 seconds) are common and generally do not require additional anti-arrhythmic treatment. Previous trials with flecainide to suppress ventricular extrasystoles and non-sustained ventricular tachycardia in the hope that it can reduce the risk of sustained ventricular tachycardia or ventricular fibrillation, in the setting of acute myocardial infarction, demonstrated increased mortality despite reduction in ventricular extrasystoles (the CAST [Cardiac Arrhythmia Suppression Trials] study). A ventricular rhythm at a rate of <100 beats/minute, termed 'idioventricular rhythm' (Figure 10.2), is

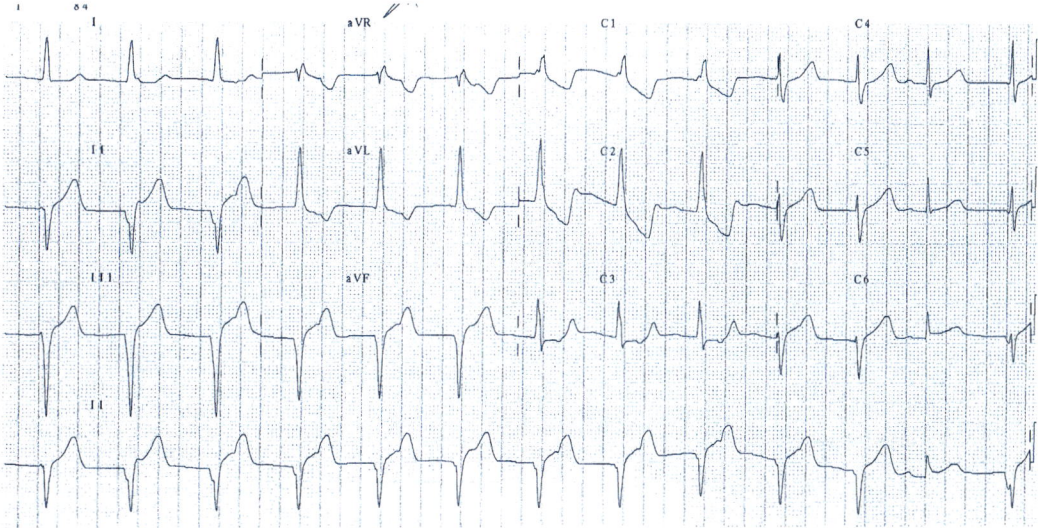

Figure 10.2 Idioventricular rhythm.

common during reperfusion therapy. This idioventricular rhythm is widely regarded as a sign of successful reperfusion, is typically asymptomatic and does not generally require treatment.

Sustained ventricular tachycardia (Figure 10.3) associated with haemodynamic compromise should be treated promptly with synchronized DC cardioversion. Patients with haemodynamically significant ventricular arrhythmia should also be treated with anti-arrhythmic agents, typically amiodarone (150–300 mg IV >30 minutes followed by 900 mg over the next 24 hours). Lignocaine is an alternative (for persistent ventricular tachycardia, 50–100 mg bolus followed by an infusion of lignocaine at 4 mg/min for the first 30 minutes, 2 mg/min for 4 hours, followed by 1 mg/min for up to 24 hours). The UK Resuscitation Council Guidelines (Figure 10.4) should be followed for a patient who has suffered a cardiac arrest.

Potential precipitants of ventricular arrhythmias should be identified and corrected (e.g. electrolyte abnormalities and pro-arrhythmic drugs). Recurrent ventricular tachycardia may be a manifestation of ongoing myocardial ischaemia and there should be a low threshold for early coronary angiography with a view to revascularization. Stent thrombosis following percutaneous coronary intervention may also present with ventricular arrhythmias and cardiac arrest and should always be considered as a potential diagnosis. An ECG following restoration of sinus rhythm may be helpful to identify ischaemia or infarction.

Ventricular tachycardia within the first 48 hours of an acute myocardial infarction is usually related to the infarction and the risk of later ventricular tachycardia is low. However, ventricular tachycardia beyond 48 hours is associated with an increased risk of future, potentially fatal, ventricular arrhythmias. In the absence of reversible causes (e.g. recurrent ischaemia or electrolyte abnormalities), these patients with sustained ventricular arrhythmia should be considered for an automated implantable cardioverter defibrillator (ICD).

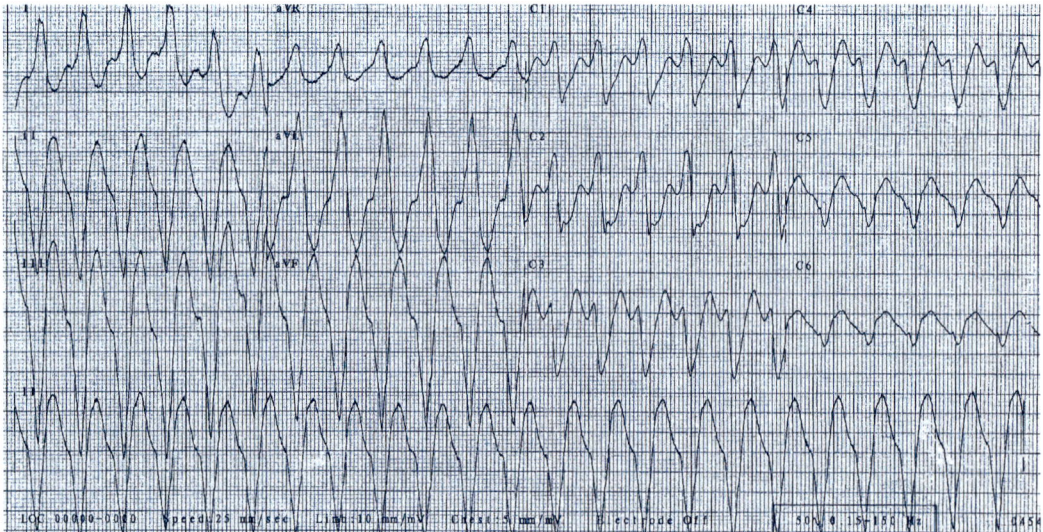

Figure 10.3 Ventricular tachycardia.

10 Peri-infarct arrhythmia

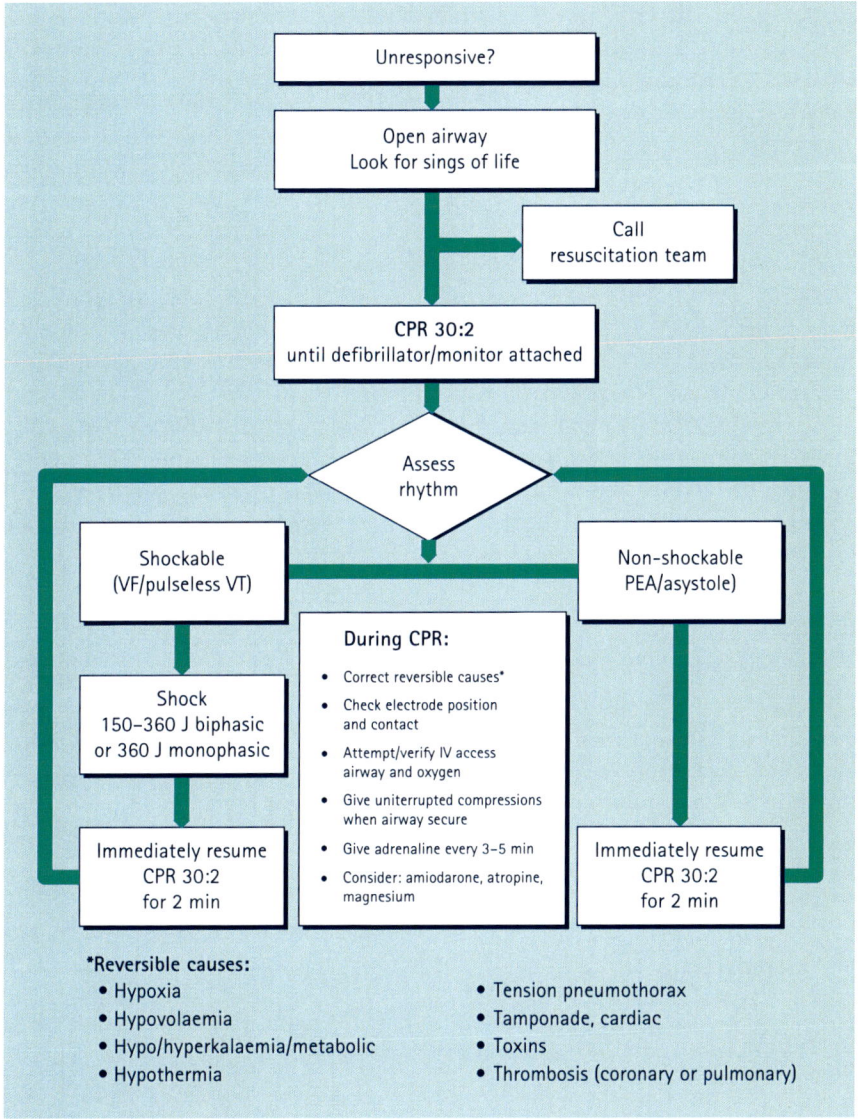

Figure 10.4 UK Resuscitation Council Guidelines for the management of a patient with cardiac arrest. PEA, pulseless electrical activity.

Supraventricular tachycardia, including atrial fibrillation and atrial flutter, are uncommon in acute myocardial infarction. The development of atrial fibrillation may signal underlying left ventricular dysfunction (and increased left ventricular filling pressure) and the development of atrial fibrillation, in turn, by increasing ventricular rate and irregularity, may exacerbate pre-existing myocardial ischaemia, reduce cardiac output and worsen cardiac failure. Hence, synchronized DC cardioversion should be considered if there is significant haemodynamic compromise, chest pain or the development of cardiac failure. If rate control is required, β-blockers may be used in the absence of pulmonary oedema or hypotension. Alternatively, amiodarone may be used if there is evidence of pulmonary oedema. Hypokalaemia and hypomagnesaemia should be corrected to maintain a serum potassium level of >4 mmol/l and magnesium level of >1 mmol/l.

Recent Developments

The early use of ICDs in patients with severe left ventricular dysfunction following myocardial infarction was tested in the DINAMIT (Defibrillator in Acute Myocardial Infarction Trial) study. Although early use of ICD (about 7 days post-infarct) reduced arrhythmic deaths, there was no reduction in overall mortality as the patients died of non-arrhythmic causes (e.g. pump failure). Based on this study, ICDs cannot be routinely recommended in the acute phase following myocardial infarctions. Of note, however, the DINAMIT study excluded patients with significant ventricular arrhythmias more than 48 hours after myocardial infarction; these patients were offered an ICD.

Conclusion

Bradyarrhythmias and tachyarrhythmias are common following acute myocardial infarction. In the context of a myocardial infarction, arrhythmias usually resolve rapidly without specific intervention. Arrhythmias may be a manifestation of myocardial ischaemia (treatment should be aimed at relieving ischaemia), may occur transiently at the time of reperfusion (usually no specific treatment is required) or may be a consequence of myocardial damage (e.g. pacemaker for complete heart block or automated ICD for late-onset ventricular arrhythmias).

Further Reading

Lim HS, Lip GY, Tse HF. Implantable cardioverter defibrillator following acute myocardial infarction: the '48-hour' and '40-day' rule. *Europace* 2008; **10**: 536–9.

Antman EM, Hand M, Armstrong PW, *et al;* 2004 Writing Committee Members, Anbe DT, Kushner FG, Ornato JP, *et al.* 2007 focused Update of the ACC/AHA 2004 Guidelines for the Management of Patients With ST-Elevation Myocardial Infarction: a report of the American College of Cardiology/American Heart Association Task Force on Practice Guidelines: developed in collaboration With the Canadian Cardiovascular Society endorsed by the American Academy of Family Physicians: 2007 Writing Group to Review New Evidence and Update the ACC/AHA 2004 Guidelines for the Management of Patients With ST-Elevation Myocardial Infarction, Writing on Behalf of the 2004 Writing Committee. *Circulation* 2008; **117**: 296–329.

11 Secondary prevention (lifestyle, risk factors and drug treatment)

Case History

A 74-year-old male patient sustained an anterior myocardial infarction (MI) that was treated with thrombolysis. He is a smoker (15 cigarettes/day), with a history of hypertension and diabetes and a body mass index (BMI) of 35 kg/m². He initially showed clinical signs of heart failure and a subsequent echocardiogram confirmed impaired left ventricle systolic function with an estimated left ventricle ejection fraction of 30%. His cholesterol on admission was 6.2 mmol/l. His electrocardiogram (ECG) shows anterior Q waves with a QRS duration of 126 ms.

How would you reduce his risk of future myocardial events and death?

What additional drug treatment has prognostic benefit?

Does coronary angiography, with a view to revascularization, have a role in this currently asymptomatic patient?

Should this patient be considered for an automated implantable cardioverter defibrillator?

Background

Patients who survive the initial ST elevation myocardial infarction (STEMI) are at 6–7% risk of death at 30 days (3–4% for a non-STEMI [NSTEMI]) and 3.2% over the subsequent 11 months (3.7% for NSTEMI). An integral part of the management of patients with ischaemic heart disease is the modification of lifestyle and risk factors (Figure 11.1).

This patient should be advised to stop smoking. The use of short-term nicotine replacement therapy, with those patients with heavy consumption (>10 cigarettes/day), improves smoking cessation success rates. Individuals should adopt a healthy diet with low levels of fat intake and increased fruit and vegetables, with moderate intake of alcohol. They should optimize their weight to achieve a BMI of <25 kg/m². Obesity is an independent risk factor for cardiovascular disease, and weight reduction in patients with ischaemic heart disease has been associated with a reduced risk of future cardiac events and death. Increased BMI is also associated with elevated blood pressure and a higher incidence of diabetes mellitus. Patients should take regular exercise with at least 30 minutes of aerobic exercise three times per week. Exercise is associated with improvements in

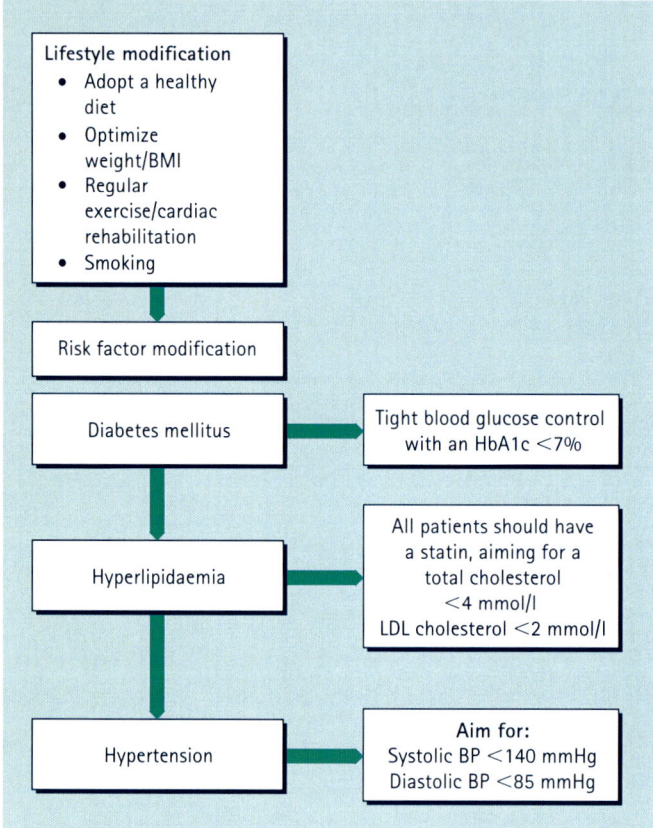

Figure 11.1 Summary of lifestyle and risk factor modification in patients with ischaemic heart disease. BMI, body mass index; BP, blood pressure; LDL, low-density lipoprotein.

blood pressure, lipid profile and reduction in weight. The majority of patients who have a MI undergo a structured programme of exercise rehabilitation, which should form part of the treatment following MI.

Approximately 20% of patients who have an acute coronary syndrome have a history of diabetes and a similar proportion may have impaired glucose tolerance. The cardiovascular benefit of glycaemic control has been debated. The DIGAMI trial (Diabetes Mellitus Insulin-Glucose Infusion in Acute Myocardial Infarction) demonstrated a reduction in mortality with aggressive glycaemic control in patients with diabetes in the 3-month period following MI. At 1 year, there was a 35% reduction in all-cause mortality. The UKPDS (United Kingdom Prospective Diabetes Study) and more recently ADVANCE (Action in Diabetes and Vascular Disease: Preterax and Diamicron Modified Release Controlled Evaluation) studies (neither a post-MI study) suggested only modest reduction in cardiovascular events with aggressive glycaemic control. In addition, data from observation studies suggest that 1% reduction in HbA1c may be associated with a 21% reduction in diabetes-related mortality and 14% reduction in MI at 10 years. Current guidelines recommend hypoglycaemic therapy to achieve an HbA1c of <7% in patients with diabetes. The glitazones (thiazolidinediones) should be avoided in patients with impaired left ventricle systolic function in NYHA (New York Heart Association) class III or IV. There have also been recent concerns about increased risk of cardiovascular events with the use of rosiglitazone.

The Joint British Societies (JBS) guidelines recommend optimization of blood pressure to 140/85 mmHg or less, with control of blood pressure being more aggressive in diabetics, or in patients with chronic renal failure, where an ideal blood pressure is <130/80 mmHg. Patients with hypertension will typically require at least two antihypertensive agents.

Elevated low-density lipoprotein cholesterol is associated with a worse outcome in patients with ischaemic heart disease. The 4S study (Scandinavian Simvastatin Survival Study) showed a 30% reduction in all-cause mortality in patients with angina or previous MI treated with simvastatin compared with placebo. More aggressive lipid-lowering therapy with high-dose atorvastatin may provide additional benefit compared with standard dose pravastatin. Hence, irrespective of baseline cholesterol level, all patients should be treated with a HMG-CoA reductase inhibitor (statin). The JBS guidelines for the management of hyperlipidaemia recommend levels of total cholesterol <4 mmol/l and low-density lipoprotein cholesterol of <2 mmol/l. A number of studies have suggested additional beneficial effects of statins on platelet adhesion, thrombosis, plaque stability, endothelial function and vascular inflammation, but the extent to which these 'pleiotropic' effects contribute to the clinical benefit is not clear. Omega-3 fatty acid, which improves several lipid parameters, has also been shown to improve outcome in patients with coronary artery disease (GISSI [Gruppo Italiano per lo Studio della Sopravvivenza nell'Infarto Miocardico)-Prevenzione] and should be considered in patients following MI.

What additional drug treatment has prognostic benefit?

Antiplatelet treatment

All patients should have lifelong aspirin therapy at 75 mg OD following a MI. Long-term aspirin use is associated with a 12% reduction in all-cause mortality and a 25% reduction in fatal and non-fatal vascular events, including MI and stroke. If aspirin is contraindicated, then clopidogrel 75 mg should be used as an alternative. Clopidogrel was shown in the CAPRIE trial (Clopidogrel versus Aspirin in Patients at Risk of Ischaemic Events) to be at least as effective as aspirin in preventing ischaemic stroke, MI and cardiovascular death in patients with atherosclerotic vascular disease. In the CURE trial (Clopidogrel in Unstable Angina to Prevent Recurrent Events), the combination of aspirin and clopidogrel 75 mg OD administered for a year following an episode of unstable angina or NSTEMI was associated with a 20% reduction in cardiovascular death, MI and stroke. The combination of aspirin and clopidogrel is generally used for 12 months following MI (particularly after coronary stenting) followed by aspirin monotherapy.

β-blockers

β-blockers result in a 24% reduction in death following an acute MI and should be given to all patients unless contraindicated. β-blockers are additionally beneficial in patients with hypertension and those with impaired left ventricular systolic function. Survival benefit has been consistently demonstrated in several large studies. Patients who have peripheral vascular disease or chronic obstructive pulmonary disease are often denied the benefits of β-blockers (40% relative risk reduction) due to perceived contraindications. However, β-blockers are not associated with a reduction in peripheral perfusion in peripheral vascular disease. Patients with chronic obstructive pulmonary disease should receive a trial of β-blockers, as the majority will tolerate the therapy without a significant reduction in peak flow.

Angiotensin-converting enzyme inhibitors

All patients should be treated with an angiotensin-converting enzyme inhibitor following a MI. Although all patients with ischaemic heart disease benefit from therapy, the greatest benefits are seen in those patients with impaired left ventricular systolic function or diabetes. Ramipril is the angiotensin-converting enzyme inhibitor of choice and this should be started at 1.25 mg OD in patients with good left ventricular systolic function and twice daily in patients with impaired left ventricular systolic function. In the EUROPA study (EUropean trial on Reduction Of cardiac events with Perindopril in stable coronary Artery disease), patients with stable coronary disease who received perindopril had a 20% reduction in cardiovascular death, MI or cardiac arrest compared with placebo. Angiotensin-converting enzyme inhibitors should be started in the first 36 hours following a MI.

Aldosterone receptor blocker

Eplerenone is an aldosterone receptor antagonist and should be started at 25 mg OD, uptitrating to 50 mg OD, in patients who have had a STEMI and have an ejection fraction of <40% and either clinical evidence of heart failure or diabetes mellitus (EPHESUS [Eplerenone Post-Acute Myocardial Infarction Heart Failure Efficacy and Survival Study]). Spironolactone improves survival in patients with class III or IV heart failure (RALES, Randomized Aldosterone Evaluation Study), but has not been studied in the early period following MI.

Does coronary angiography, with a view to revascularization, have a role in this currently asymptomatic patient?

All patients who develop an acute coronary syndrome should be considered for coronary angiography with a view to revascularization of the culprit vessel deemed responsible for the acute coronary syndrome, irrespective of whether the patient's symptoms have stabilized following the initial myocardial event.

In contrast to elective angioplasty for patients with stable coronary artery disease, coronary angioplasty (and stenting) in the context of a MI has been shown to reduce the risk of subsequent myocardial ischaemic events. In the FRISC II study (Fragmin during Instability in Coronary Artery Disease II), an early invasive strategy in patients with unstable angina was associated with a significant reduction in death, MI, the need for readmission and the need for revascularization in the first year. There was also a significant reduction in death and MI at 6 months follow-up in patients with NSTEMI.

Patients with severe coronary artery disease benefit prognostically from coronary artery bypass graft surgery. This includes patients with three-vessel coronary artery disease, significant left main stem coronary artery disease (>50%) and proximal two-vessel disease, including proximal left anterior descending artery. Patients with additional impaired left ventricular systolic function or diabetes mellitus particularly benefit from coronary artery bypass graft surgery.

Should this patient be considered for an automated implantable cardioverter defibrillator?

Sudden arrhythmic death is a common cause of mortality in patients who have survived an acute MI. Ventricular arrhythmias may occur months or even years after the initial MI and are believed to be related to scarring of the myocardium. Implantable cardioverter defibrillators (ICD) should be considered in patients with a history of MI for primary prevention against arrhythmic death. Current recommendations by the National Institute of Clinical Excellence 2006 guidelines for ICDs are outlined in Figure 11.2. This patient has an ejection fraction of 30% and prolongation of the QRS duration at 126 ms following his MI. Hence, he should be offered an ICD in the absence of any improvement 4 weeks after his MI (left ventricular function may improve following MI as stunned myocardium regains function).

Primary prevention (prevention of a first life-theatening arrhythmic event) for patients who have a history of previous (more than 4 weeks) myocardial infarction (MI) and:
either
– left ventricular dysfunction with a left ventricular ejection fraction (LVEF) of less than 35% (no worse than class III of the New York Heart Association functional classification of heart failure)
and
– non-sustained ventricular tachycardia (VT) on Holter (24-hour electrocardiogram [ECG]) monitoring
and
– inducible VT on electrophysiological (EP) testing
Or
– left ventricular dysfunction with an LVEF of less than 30% (no worse than class III of the New York Heart Association functional classification of heart failure)
and
– QRS duration of equal to or more than 120 milliseconds

Secondary prevention (prevention of an additional life-threatening event in survivors of sudden cardiac events or in patients with recurrent unstable rhythms for patients who present, in the absence of a treatable cause) in patients with one of the following:
- having survived a cardiac arrest due to either VT or ventricular fibrillation
- spontaneous sustained VT causing syncope or significant haemodynamic compromise
- sustained VT without syncope or cardiac arrest, and who have an associated reduction in ejection fraction (LVEF of less than 35%) (no worse than class III of the New York Heart Association functional classification of heart failure).

Figure 11.2 National Institute for Health and Clinical Excellence 2006 guidelines for automatic implantable cardioverter defibrillators in the context of ischaemic heart disease.

Recent Developments

Increased oxidative stress and homocysteine levels have been associated with coronary artery disease. On this basis, vitamins (antioxidants) and folic acid (lowers homocysteine) were believed to be beneficial. However, a number of placebo-controlled randomized trials (and subsequent systematic reviews and meta-analysis) of vitamins and folic acid supplementation failed to demonstrate any benefit in the setting of primary or secondary prevention. Hence, vitamin and folic acid supplementation is not recommended following acute coronary syndromes.

Conclusion

Aggressive risk factor management has been shown to reduce future cardiovascular events. All patients should therefore be offered comprehensive risk factor management following MI, which will typically include lipid-lowering therapy (statin), antihypertensive agents and antiplatelet therapy. ICDs may reduce the risk of sudden arrhythmic death in some patients with impaired left ventricular function.

Further Reading

JBS 2: Joint British Societies' guidelines on prevention of cardiovascular disease in clinical practice. *Heart* 2005; **91**: 1–52.

Acknowledgement

The authors warmly acknowledge the contribution of Dr J Khan, Consultant Cardiologist, Sandwell and West Birmingham NHS Trust, UK, to chapters 4–11 of this book.

SECTION THREE   03

Arterial Disease and Syncope

12	Aortic dissection
13	Hypertensive emergencies
14	Neurocardiogenic syncope
15	Cardiac tumours

PROBLEM

12 Aortic dissection

Case History

A 56-year-old woman presented to the emergency department with sudden-onset severe central chest pain that radiated to her neck. She had never had chest pains as severe as this before. She smokes 20 cigarettes a day and has a history of hypertension. She takes ramipril normally for her hypertension. At presentation, she was clearly distressed with severe chest pain. Her blood pressure in her right arm was 118/70 mmHg and the blood pressure in her left arm was comparable. Her heart rate was 104 beats/minute and oxygen saturation was 98% on air. Her heart sounds were normal. Her electrocardiogram showed sinus tachycardia but not ST segment shift. Her chest X-ray was normal. During her clinical assessment, she was noted to have intermittent weakness, particularly on her right side and the astute physician noted loud left-sided carotid bruit.

What is the possible diagnosis?

How would you confirm the diagnosis?

How would you manage this patient?

Background

Chest pain may be cardiac (e.g. myocardial ischaemia/infarction, pericarditis), pulmonary (e.g. pulmonary embolism, pneumothorax), gastrointestinal (e.g. oesophageal spasm, oesophagitis) or musculoskeletal in origin. Aortic dissection is an uncommon but potentially fatal cause of chest pain. In this case, the neurological symptoms and carotid bruit in association with her chest pain without evidence of ischaemia should raise the suspicion of aortic dissection. The normal chest X-ray and the absence of significant blood pressure difference between the right and left arm should not detract the physician from making the diagnosis, as widened mediastinum and pulse deficit may be absent in over one-third and two-thirds of patients respectively (Table 12.1). Aortic dissection is often associated with atherosclerotic cardiovascular disease and hypertension, which may steer the unwary physician towards the diagnosis of acute coronary syndrome. Hence, a high level of clinical suspicion is essential.

Table 12.1 Clinical presentation of aortic dissection

	Type A	Type B	Overall
Symptoms and signs			
Severe chest/back pain	85%	86%	85%
Worst ever pain	90%	90%	90%
Abrupt onset	91%	89%	90%
Abdominal pain	22%	43%	30%
Pulse deficit	31%	21%	27%
Aortic regurgitation	44%	12%	32%
Chest X-ray			
Widened mediastinum	63%	56%	60%
Normal	11%	21%	16%
Electrocardiogram			
Normal	30%	31%	30%

How would you confirm the diagnosis?

Transoesophageal echocardiography, computed tomographic (CT) angiography and magnetic resonance imaging (MRI) have all shown a sensitivity and specificity of over 95%. As CT angiography is widely available and can provide important information to guide treatment, it is generally the first choice in most centres. Important information relevant to the management of a patient with aortic dissection includes the extent of dissection, localization of intimal tear, size of the true and false lumen, involvement and perfusion of aortic branches (either by true or false lumen), possible aortic valve involvement proximally, and presence of haematoma and effusion. Transthoracic echocardiography can sometimes visualize the dissection flap (proximal aortic dissection) and assess the presence/severity of aortic dissection and pericardial effusion.

There are different classifications for aortic dissection. The widely used Stanford classification divides aortic dissection into types A and B. Type A refers to any dissection that involves the ascending aorta and in type B the ascending aorta is not affected. The De Bakey classification makes a further distinction for aortic dissection affecting the length of the aorta. The Svensson classification is a pathological classification (Table 12.2). The Stanford classification is widely used due to its simplicity and implications for treatment.

The complications of aortic dissection are related to the involvement of aortic branches and the integrity of the aortic wall. Hence, myocardial ischaemia and infarction (coronary arteries), upper limb ischaemia (subclavian arteries), cerebral ischaemia and

Table 12.2 Classification of aortic dissection

Stanford classification
  Type A: any involvement of ascending aorta
  Type B: no involvement of ascending aorta

De Bakey classification
  Type 1: entire length affected
  Type 2: ascending aorta affected
  Type 3: descending aorta affected

Svensson classification
  Class 1: dissection with true and false lumen
  Class 2: intramural haematoma
  Class 3: subtle dissection without haematoma
  Class 4: atherosclerotic penetrating ulcer
  Class 5: traumatic dissection (including iatrogenic causes)

stroke (carotid and vertebral arteries), spinal cord ischaemia (lumbar arteries), abdominal visceral ischaemia (coeliac and mesenteric arteries), renal failure (renal arteries) and lower limb ischaemia (iliac arteries) are all recognized complications of aortic dissection, either as a result of avulsion or thrombosis of the artery. Proximally, involvement of the aortic valve can result in catastrophic aortic regurgitation and heart failure. Haemorrhagic pericardial effusion and tamponade may occur. Some of these potential complications of aortic dissection are shown in Figure 12.1. In this case, the patient underwent a CT scan that confirmed an extensive aortic dissection involving the proximal and distal aorta (Stanford type A). The transthoracic echocardiogram did not show any aortic regurgitation of pericardial effusion.

How would you manage this patient?

Management is dependent on the type and complications associated with the aortic dissection (Figure 12.2). Type B dissections are usually managed medically with tight

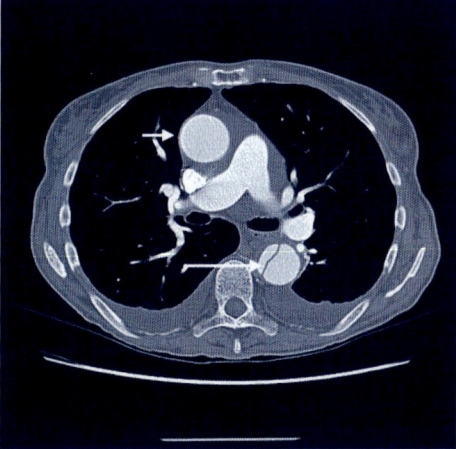

Figure 12.1 Computed tomography scan demonstrating a dissection flap in the descending aorta (long arrow). There is no dissection in the ascending aorta (short arrow).

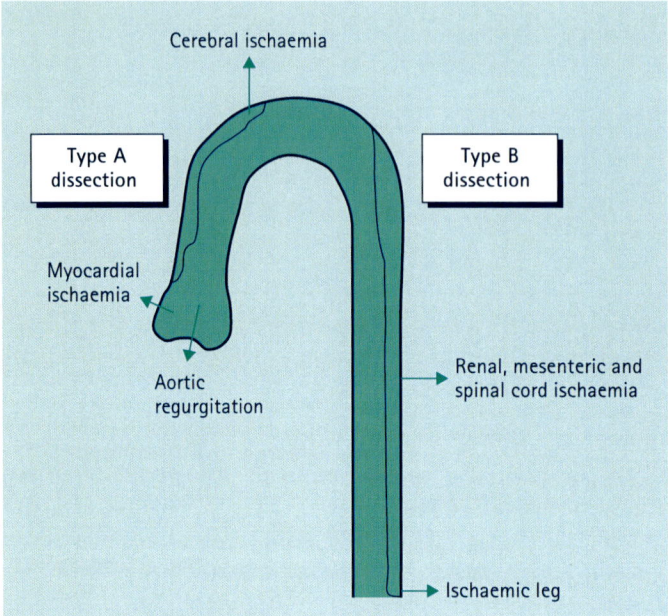

Figure 12.2 Complications of aortic dissection.

control of the blood pressure (systolic blood pressure of 100–120 mmHg) with negatively inotropic agents (e.g. β-blockers or verapamil if β-blockers are contraindicated). Reduction in cardiac contractility is believed to reduce the shearing forces on the aorta and reduce progression of dissection or rupture. Vasodilators such as sodium nitroprusside may be added if blood pressure remains significantly elevated. Although there are no randomized studies, surgical intervention may be considered in patients with evidence of impending rupture or severe ischaemia of the abdominal viscera and lower limbs. The use of an endovascular stent graft to cover the dissection is under investigation. Adequate analgesia is essential.

Type A dissection should be treated surgically unless the patient's comorbidities are prohibitive (Figure 12.3). Medical treatment of type A dissection has a mortality rate of 50% at 30 days, compared with about 25% in surgically treated patients. The mortality may be even lower in surgically treated patients in the absence of haemodynamic compromise or significant organ ischaemia. The surgical approach is variable and complex, depending on the pathological condition, the extent of dissection, involvement of coronary arteries or aortic valves and the experience/preferences of the surgeon. In general, the affected segment of ascending aorta/arch is resected and replaced with a prosthetic graft. The aortic valve and the coronary arteries may need to be replaced or reconstructed if affected. Preservation of the aortic valve will obviate the need for anticoagulation but is associated with the need for reoperation. The approach to repair of the descending aorta in the case of extensive aortic dissection is controversial and a combined approach with endovascular stent placement has been suggested.

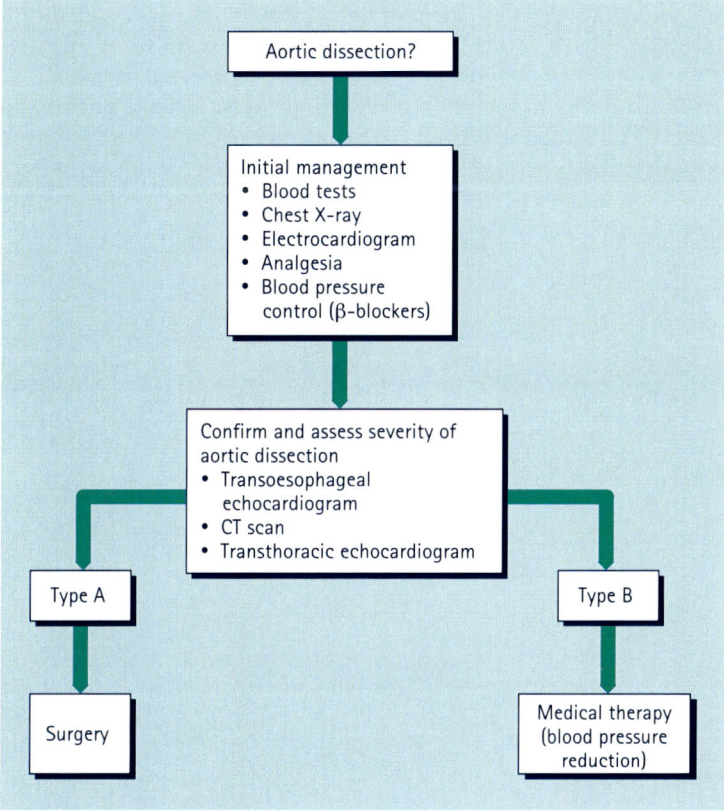

Figure 12.3 Management of aortic dissection.

Recent Developments

 Percutaneous techniques using endovascular stents have been studied over the last few years. In type A dissection, the extensive resection of the distal aorta may be associated with increased morbidity and mortality. Endovascular stenting has been used in combination with surgical repair of type A dissection to limit resection of aorta. Endovascular stents have also been used to treat distal type B dissection, although early data from the INSTEAD study (INvestigation of STEnt Grafts in Patients with Type B Aortic Dissection) indicated equivalent mortality in patients with type B dissection treated medically with or without endovascular stenting with covered stents.

Conclusion

 The diagnosis of aortic dissection requires a high level of clinical suspicion. Diagnosis can often be confirmed by transoesophageal echocardiogram or CT angiography. Dissection involving the ascending aorta (Stanford type A) should be treated by urgent surgery, usually with replacement of the affected segment by a prosthetic graft. A type B dissection (i.e. ascending aorta not affected) may be managed medically with control of blood pressure. β-blockers are the recommended first-line agents for blood pressure control.

Further Reading

Golledge J, Eagle KA. Acute aortic dissection. *Lancet* 2008; **372**: 55–66.

PROBLEM

13 Hypertensive emergencies

Case History

A 60-year-old man presented to his general practitioner for a routine cardiovascular assessment, as he was concerned about his risk of a heart attack. He is a builder and smokes about 10 cigarettes a day. He had never seen his doctor previously and as such had no known history of diabetes mellitus, hypertension or hypercholesterolaemia. He does not take any regular medications and denied illicit drug use. On examination, his blood pressure was markedly elevated at 196/122 mmHg with a heart rate of 76 beats/minute. Cardiovascular examination was unremarkable.

How would you assess this patient?

How would you treat this man?

Background

This patient has markedly elevated blood pressure but has no obvious symptoms. Nonetheless, the patient should be carefully assessed for evidence of target organ damage (retinal haemorrhage and papilloedema, haematuria, encephalopathy, myocardial ischaemia or heart failure). Presence of target organ damage with severe hypertension represents a hypertensive emergency (Table 13.1). Hence, clinical assessment should include careful cardiovascular and neurological examination (including the fundus). In the absence of any evidence of target organ damage, severe hypertension (generally regarded as >180/120 mmHg) can be categorized as hypertensive urgency.

Investigations are aimed at identifying potential secondary causes of hypertension and any evidence of target organ damage. Hence, urinanalysis (e.g. haematuria and proteinuria) and blood count (e.g. haemolysis) and electrolytes (e.g. worsening renal function

Table 13.1 Hypertensive emergencies

Hypertensive encephalopathy (decreased consciousness, seizure or focal neurological deficit after excluding other intracranial pathology)

Acute target organ damage:
- aortic dissection
- acute coronary syndrome
- acute pulmonary oedema
- acute cerebral infarction
- intracranial haemorrhage
- acute or rapidly worsening renal failure

Phaeochromocytoma crisis

Guillain–Barré syndrome

Drug-related hypertension (e.g. cocaine and sympathomimetics)

Eclampsia

Microangiopathic haemolysis

and serum potassium) should be routine. A sample for plasma renin activity and aldosterone may be useful for the diagnosis of mineralocorticoid excess, and catecholamines for the diagnosis of phaeochromocytoma.

Electrocardiogram (ECG) may reveal left ventricular hypertrophy or changes suggestive of myocardial ischaemia. Chest X-rays may show evidence of cardiomegaly or pulmonary congestion. Depending on the clinical presentation, cardiac enzymes, computed tomography (CT) and/or magnetic resonance imaging (MRI) of the brain, thorax or abdomen may also be indicated (e.g. intracranial bleed or aortic dissection). In this case, the patient was admitted to hospital. Cardiovascular and neurological examination was normal. Fundoscopy showed arteriovenous nipping consistent with hypertension but no haemorrhage or papilloedema. (The grading of retinopathy is listed in Table 13.2.) ECG showed left ventricular hypertrophy but chest X-ray was unremarkable. Urinalysis, blood count and electrolytes were also normal. This man has no clinical evidence of target organ damage. Therefore, this man has hypertensive urgency.

Table 13.2 Keith–Wagner classification of retinopathy

Grade 1	Mild arteriolar narrowing or sclerosis
Grade 2	Arteriovenous nipping and marked sclerosis of arterioles
Grade 3	Retinal haemorrhages, exudates and cotton wool spots (ischaemia)
Grade 4	Grade 3 plus papilloedema

How would you treat this man?

Hypertensive urgency does not require emergency intravenous antihypertensive therapy. Indeed, rapid blood pressure reduction may have detrimental effects. Oral antihypertensive therapy, such as amlodipine, may be a reasonable choice with the aim of reducing the blood pressure gradually over 24–48 hours. An oral β-blocker or angiotensin-converting enzyme inhibitor might be a reasonable alternative. Sublingual nifedipine, with unpredictable blood pressure-lowering effects should be avoided. Hospital admission is not mandatory if appropriate close outpatient monitoring of therapy is available.

The treatment of hypertensive emergency is dependent on the nature of the target organ damage (Figure 13.1). Parenteral therapy is generally recommended in patients with hypertensive emergencies. Parenteral antihypertensive agents are listed in Table 13.3. Sodium nitroprusside is a potent, short-acting arteriolar and venous dilator, and may be used in most hypertensive emergencies. However, blood pressure should be closely monitored (with arterial line) and prolonged use should be avoided in view of the risk of cyanate toxicity (increasing metabolic acidosis, abnormal respiratory pattern and

Table 13.3 Parenteral antihypertensive agents

Drug	Dose	Duration	Side effects
Sodium nitroprusside	0.25–10 µg/kg/min	1–2 min	Hypotension, cyanate toxicity
Labetolol	20–80 mg bolus 1–2 mg/min infusion	2–6 h	Bronchospasm, heart block
Glyceryl trinitrate	5–100 µg/min	5–15 min	Headache
Furosemide	40–80 mg	2 h	Hypotension
Hydralazine	10–20 mg bolus	2–6 h	Reflex tachycardia
Phentolamine	5–10 mg bolus	3–5 min	Reflex tachycardia

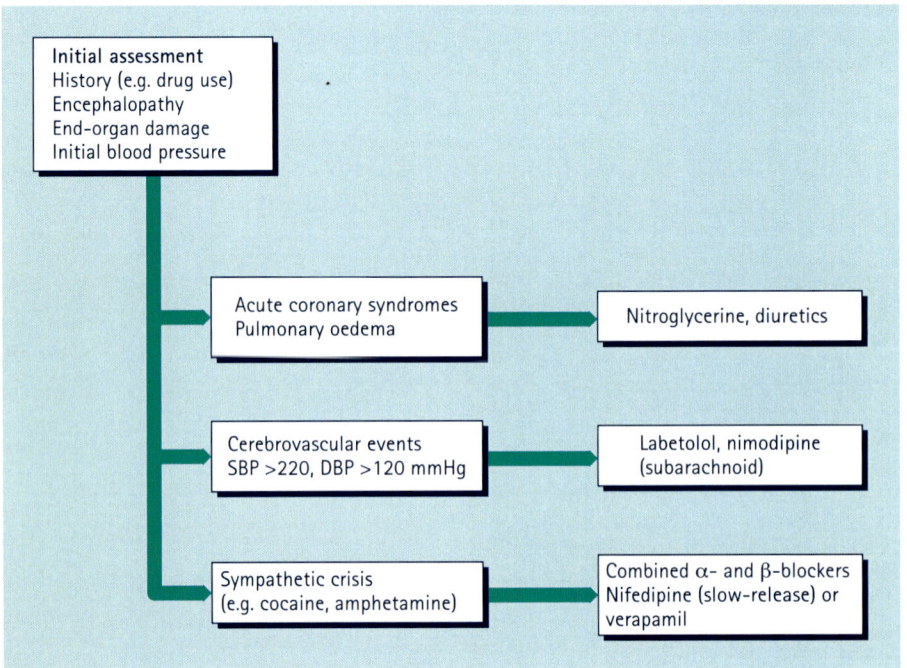

Figure 13.1 Management of hypertensive emergencies.

deterioration in consciousness), particularly with renal or hepatic dysfunction. Labetolol, which has α- and β-adrenergic-blocking properties is also an appropriate antihypertensive therapy in most hypertensive emergencies.

Cardiac ischaemia may be appropriately treated with intravenous nitrates and β-blocker therapy. Intravenous nitrates are also appropriate for heart failure (with the addition of sodium nitroprusside if required). The treatment of hypertension in aortic dissection should include a β-blocker to reduce the contractility and potential shearing forces on the dissection flap (e.g. intravenous labetolol). This may be combined with a vasodilator (e.g. sodium nitroprusside or nitrates). Hypertensive emergencies in the setting of phaeochromocytoma or catecholamine excess (e.g. cocaine or tyramine crisis) should always include an α-adrenergic blocker (e.g. intravenous phentolamine) in addition to a β-adrenergic blocker, as a β-blocker in isolation will result in unopposed α-adrenergic-mediated vasoconstriction and greater blood pressure rise. Indeed, α-blockade should precede β-blocker therapy.

The treatment of hypertension in acute stroke is controversial. Blood pressure-lowering therapy is generally recommended if blood pressure exceeds 220/120 mmHg. Treatment may be initiated with intravenous labetolol, with the addition of nitrates or nitroprusside if needed, and titrated cautiously to obtain an initial reduction in blood pressure of about 10–15%. Antihypertensive therapy may be initiated in patients with blood pressure exceeding 180/110 mmHg if associated with intracranial haemorrhage or stroke treated with thrombolysis.

Finally, it should be noted that long-term blood pressure control is mandatory in patients with hypertensive emergencies or urgencies. Non-compliance with antihypertensive therapy is a major cause of hypertensive urgencies and emergencies. In this case, the patient was commenced on amlodipine and discharged the next day following minor reductions in blood pressure to 182/116 mmHg.

Recent Developments

Recent data from one of the largest series of patients with hypertensive emergencies suggest that survival in patients presenting with hypertensive emergencies, previously known as malignant hypertension, has improved over the last three decades. This is largely due to better control of blood pressure and management of cardiovascular risk. Renal impairment at presentation does not necessarily indicate permanent renal failure and may improve with blood pressure control in a large proportion of cases.

Conclusion

A patient with severe hypertension should be carefully evaluated for evidence of target organ damage. The presence of target organ damage distinguishes hypertensive emergencies from hypertensive urgencies. The latter should be managed with oral antihypertensive therapy with a gradual blood pressure reduction over days. Treatment of hypertensive emergencies is dependent on the nature of the target organ damage. In general, rapid blood pressure reduction should be avoided.

Further Reading

Marik PE, Varon J. Hypertensive crises: challenges and management. *Chest* 2007; **131**: 1949–62.

PROBLEM

14 Neurocardiogenic syncope

Case History

A 32-year-old woman was brought into the emergency department following an episode of transient loss of consciousness. She described a sensation of nausea, sweatiness, and light-headedness about half a minute prior to the loss of consciousness. She works as a secretary and was standing in a queue at that time. She believed that she did not lose consciousness for more than a minute or so. She did not suffer any injuries and denied loss of continence during the event. She recovered within a few minutes. She has not had similar episodes prior to this. She has no other medical history of note and does not take any regular medications. Cardiovascular examination was normal.

What are the causes of syncope and what is the likely diagnosis?

How would you investigate this patient?

How would you treat this patient?

Background

Syncope refers to a transient loss of consciousness and must be differentiated from non-syncopal attacks (Table 14.1). Contrary to widely held beliefs, transient ischaemic attacks of the anterior circulation (i.e. carotid artery territory) do not usually cause syncope and must be distinguished from true syncope. True syncopal episodes are most commonly caused by neurally mediated reflex, of which vasovagal syncope is the most common. The 'vagal' effects usually include gastrointestinal, respiratory and cardiac symptoms, which are typically precipitated by prolonged standing in crowded places, following a meal, post-exercise, or sudden exposure to pain. Importantly, cardiac disease can cause syncopal episodes. Unlike syncope without structural heart disease, patients with syncope associated with cardiac disease have worse outcomes and should be appropriately investigated and treated. In this case, the patient gives a typical history of vasovagal syncope with prodromal symptoms.

14 Neurocardiogenic syncope

Table 14.1 Causes of syncopal and non-syncopal episodes

Syncope	Non-syncopal episodes
Neurally mediated • Vasovagal • Carotid sinus hypersensitivity • Situational syncope (e.g. post-exercise, postprandial, cough)	**No loss of consciousness** • Falls • Cataplexy • Transient ischaemic attack • Psychogenic
Orthostatic hypotension • Autonomic failure (primary: multisystem atrophy, pure autonomic failure; secondary: diabetic or amyloid neuropathy) • Drugs • Volume depletion • Metabolic (e.g. hypoglycaemia)	**Partial/complete loss of consciousness** • Epilepsy • Intoxication • Vertebrobasilar ischaemia
Cardiac arrhythmias (e.g. sinus node dysfunction, heart block, ventricular arrhythmia)	
Structural cardiopulmonary disease (e.g. aortic stenosis, pulmonary embolism, aortic dissection)	
Cerebrovascular	
Subclavian steal syndrome	

- Syncope during exercise should not be considered neurally mediated syncope. Structural heart disease should be excluded in these patients.
- Cerebral ischaemia of the carotid artery territory does not usually cause syncope. Subclavian steal refers to reduction in vertebral artery circulation and compromised posterior circulation with arm exercise.

How would you investigate this patient?

The European Society of Cardiology has issued guidelines on the assessment of patients with syncope. The EGSYS study (Evaluation of Guidelines in Syncope Study) of consecutive patients referred to the syncope service suggests good diagnostic yield (diagnosis in 98% of cases) and even reduced hospital admissions with adherence to these guidelines. Based on these guidelines, the initial assessment should include a detailed history (including witness accounts) and examination, supine and upright blood pressures and a standard 12-lead electrocardiogram (ECG). Based on these assessments, true syncopal events should be differentiated from non-syncopal events. The diagnosis of vasovagal syncope based on these initial assessments may be sufficiently certain (as in this case) and if isolated or occuring only rarely, generally does not require further investigations.

Patients with true syncope of uncertain diagnosis and suggestive evidence of cardiac disease (e.g. based on ECG) should undergo further cardiac evaluations, which may include echocardiogram, prolonged ambulatory ECG recording, stress testing and electrophysiological testing. In the absence of structural heart disease, patients should undergo neurally mediated tests, which usually include head-up tilt testing, carotid sinus massage and ambulatory ECG monitoring (Figure 14.1). An implantable loop recorder (implanted subcutaneously) allows prolonged monitoring (>18 months) and may improve the diagnostic yield and should be considered in patients with recurrent episodes (>3 episodes in 2 years) affecting quality of life or at high risk of injury (e.g. no warning symptoms or high-risk occupation).

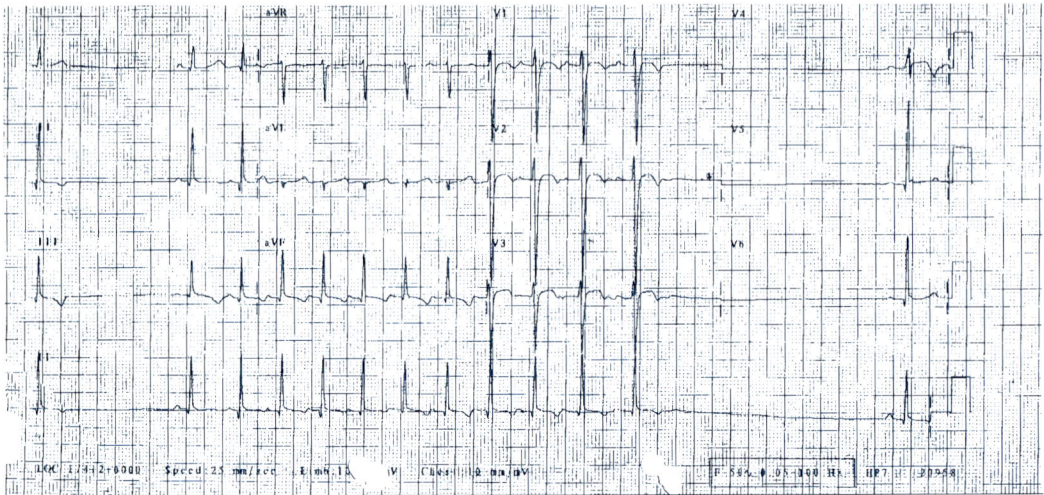

Figure 14.1 Sinus pause following brief supraventricular tachycardia. The prolonged recovery of sinus node function is typical of sinus node disease. Syncope is more likely to be related to the sinus pause, rather than the tachycardia.

How would you treat this patient?

Treatment of syncope should be targeted at the cause. For example, orthostatic hypotension due to overenthusiastic use of vasodilators may be corrected by withdrawal of treatment; cardiac arrhythmias such as ventricular tachycardia or sinus node disease (Figure 14.2) or complete heart block may require an implantable defibrillator or permanent pacemaker, and structural heart disease may require surgical treatment.

The majority of cases of vasovagal syncope tend to be isolated events (as in this case) or to reoccur only rarely. Longitudinal studies suggest that vasovagal syncope in young patients has a benign prognosis and in many cases, improves with age. The prognosis in the elderly may be worse, but this may be related to greater comorbidities. Hence, young patients may be reassured and offered advice about maintaining adequate hydration and avoiding potential precipitants (e.g. prolonged standing). Tilt training and the use of compression stockings have been advocated but generally uptake and compliance are unsatisfactory. This case was managed conservatively with simple lifestyle advice.

Patients with recurrent vasovagal syncope may require treatment. A number of pharmacological treatments have been studied in vasovagal syncope, such as β-blockers, disopyramide, selective serotonin reuptake inhibitors (e.g. fluoxetine), fludrocortisone and vasoconstrictors (e.g. midodrine). In general, small observational studies suggest benefit but these treatments have either yet to be formally tested in larger randomized studies or randomized trials to date have failed to confirm their benefit in vasovagal syncope. In particular, β-blockers were widely used in vasovagal syncope, but the recent POST study (Prevention of Syncope Trial) of 208 patients with syncope and positive head-up tilt test (metoprolol versus placebo) failed to demonstrate a reduction in syncopal episodes. Furthermore, a number of these medications may result in significant adverse effects and discontinuation of treatment in 25–30% of patients in a year. Vasoconstrictors can cause hypertension, urinary frequency and exacerbation of ischaemic heart disease. Fludrocortisone can cause hypertension and oedema and one

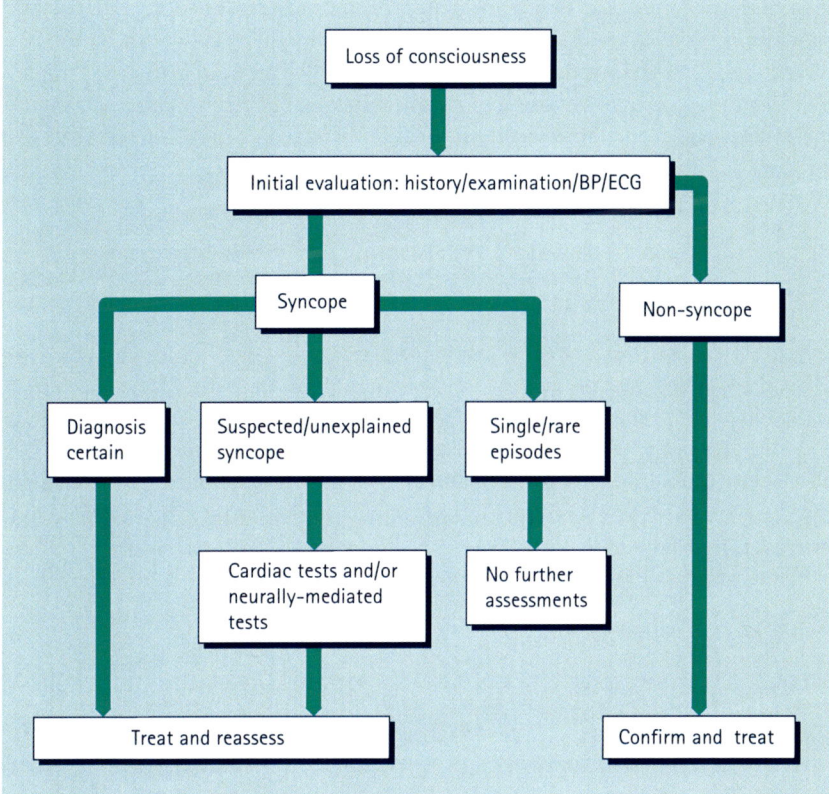

Figure 14.2 Assessment of loss of consciousness. BP, blood pressure.

study even suggested worse outcome when compared with placebo. Disopyramide has significant antimuscarinic effects (e.g. dry eyes, dry mouth and urinary retention).

The failure of medical treatment and the frequent observation of bradycardia and asystole in patients with syncope prompted studies into the use of permanent pacemakers. Early (non-placebo-controlled) small studies suggested significant reductions in syncopal episodes, but more recently two randomized placebo-controlled trials (VPS (Vasovagal Pacemaker Study) II and SYNPACE (SYNcope and PACing)) have failed to reproduce the promising results of earlier studies. It is increasingly clear that positive tilt testing identifies a heterogeneous patient population with variable mechanisms of syncope (only about 50% may be related to bradycardia/asystole). As pacemakers can only prevent syncope due to bradycardia/asystole, it is not surprising that these randomized trials, which included unselected patients with a positive tilt test, failed to show significant benefit.

This major limitation of tilt testing has led to greater use of implantable loop recorders to document the presence of bradycardia/asystole in association with syncope, which might benefit from a permanent pacemaker. The use of implantable loop recorders is associated with greater diagnostic yield, and the ISSUE 2 study (International Study on Syncope of Uncertain Etiology 2) suggests that treatment guided by the findings of an implantable loop recorder (e.g. pacemaker for bradycardia/asystole and catheter ablation for arrhythmia) can significantly reduce the recurrence of syncope (about 80% relative risk reduction). More importantly, the approach of delaying treatment until documentation of bradycardia/asystole by the implantable loop recorder appears to be safe. Hence, implantable loop recorders should be considered in patients with neurally mediated syncope, particularly in high-risk patients (e.g. recurrent syncope, significant injuries due to syncope or high-risk occupation).

Recent Developments

The value of tilt testing has been challenged by a number of clinical studies, which suggested a lack of correlation between the results of the tilt test and the mechanism of syncope documented by implantable loop recorders. Hence, some patients with asystole on tilt testing may not have significant changes in heart rate during syncope, while some patients with a vasodepressor response on tilt testing, generally believed to be unsuitable for pacemaker therapy, may develop asystole during syncope. The response to tilt testing may therefore not be useful in guiding specific therapy. Future studies will further evaluate the use of implantable loop recorders in guiding treatment for syncope.

Conclusion

Syncope refers to a transient loss of consciousness and should be distinguished from non-syncopal episodes. Syncope is most commonly neurally mediated, vasovagal syncope being the most common. Other differential diagnoses include orthostatic hypotension, arrhythmias and cardiopulmonary disease. ECG, echocardiography and ambulatory monitoring may be useful for excluding structural heart disease. Vasovagal syncope in the young has a benign prognosis and patients should be reassured. Simple lifestyle measures may be adequate but in some cases with documented bradycardia/asystole, permanent pacemakers may reduce the recurrence of syncope. Implantable loop recorders should be considered in the assessment of patients with recurrent or high-risk neurally mediated syncope.

Further Reading

Brignole M. Diagnosis and treatment of syncope. *Heart* 2007; **93**: 130–6.

Brignole M, Sutton R, Menozzi C, *et al.* Early application of an implantable loop recorder allows effective specific therapy in patients with recurrent suspected neurally mediated syncope. *Eur Heart J* 2006; **27**: 1085–92.

PROBLEM

15 Cardiac tumours

Case History

A 56-year-old woman presented with 2 days of pre-syncopal symptoms against a background of breathlessness on exertion over the last week. She had been feeling generally lethargic with weight loss of about 4 kg over the last few months. She had been diagnosed with hypertension and commenced on bendroflumethiazide about 3 months previously and thought her symptoms were related to the medication. She has no known cardiac or respiratory disease and no history of rheumatic fever. She is a non-smoker. On examination, her blood pressure was 142/80 mmHg with a heart rate of 84 beats/minute. There was an audible diastolic murmur but heart sounds were normal otherwise. Her chest was clear. There was only minimal peripheral oedema.

What are the causes of diastolic murmurs?

How would you investigate this patient?

What are the clinical features of cardiac myxomas?

What are the other types of neoplasms of the heart?

How would you manage cardiac myxomas?

Background

Murmurs in diastole are generally classified into either early or mid/late diastolic murmurs. Early diastolic murmurs are usually related to aortic regurgitation and less commonly pulmonary regurgitation secondary to pulmonary hypertension (Graham–Steell murmur). The murmur associated with chronic severe aortic regurgitation is typically long (as the left ventricular compliance increases to accommodate the increased volume load) with a high frequency blowing character. In contrast, the early diastolic murmur of acute aortic regurgitation may be brief as pressure rapidly equilibrates in the non-compliant left ventricle.

Mid-diastolic murmurs are usually caused by mitral stenosis and less commonly tricuspid regurgitation. The latter, as in other murmurs originating from the right side of the heart typically increases in intensity with inspiration (increased venous return and blood flow in the right side of the heart). Rarely, atrial myxoma may result in obstruction of the mitral or tricuspid valve and generate a diastolic murmur. A 'tumour plop' may be mistaken as the second heart sound.

How would you investigate this patient?

Diastolic murmurs should be considered pathological and deserve further investigation, particularly if the patient is symptomatic. Transthoracic echocardiography is a useful first-line investigation. In this case, the transthoracic echocardiogram showed a round mobile mass in the left atrium, which appeared to arise from the atrial septum and extend towards the mitral valve (Figure 15.1). The left atrium was mildly dilated and left ventricular function was normal. There were no other abnormalities. The appearance was suggestive of an atrial myxoma.

What are the clinical features of cardiac myxomas?

Cardiac myxomas are the commonest primary cardiac neoplasms in adults and affect women more commonly than men. They are usually diagnosed in the fifth or sixth decade of life. The majority of cardiac myxomas are found in the atria (75% in the left atrium), arising from the fossa ovalis of the atrial septum, with a broad base or sometimes a narrow pedicle. The mass itself is variable, and can be soft, friable or firm, cystic, haemorrhagic, calcified or even ossified. The identification of myxoma cells allows histological diagnosis of myxoma. Cardiac myxomas may also be multiple, familial and can present as part of a clinical syndrome (with neurofibromas, naevi and lentigines) related to germ-line mutations.

Like many other neoplasms, atrial myxomas may present with vague systemic symptoms of lethargy, fever, arthralgia and weight loss, and mimic infective illnesses (e.g. endocarditis). Atrial myxomas may obstruct blood flow from the atrium to the ventricle (a ball valve effect), which may result in pulmonary congestion, progressive heart failure, pulmonary oedema, haemoptysis, syncope and chest tightness simulating angina. Systemic embolism is also well described in patients with atrial myxomas. Cardiac myxomas may present with any or all of this triad of symptoms, i.e. constitutional, obstructive or embolic symptoms, but may also be asymptomatic.

What are the other types of neoplasms of the heart?

Cardiac tumours are generally quite rare (0.03% on autopsy) and may be primary or secondary (i.e. metastatic); the former may be benign or malignant. The majority (75%) of

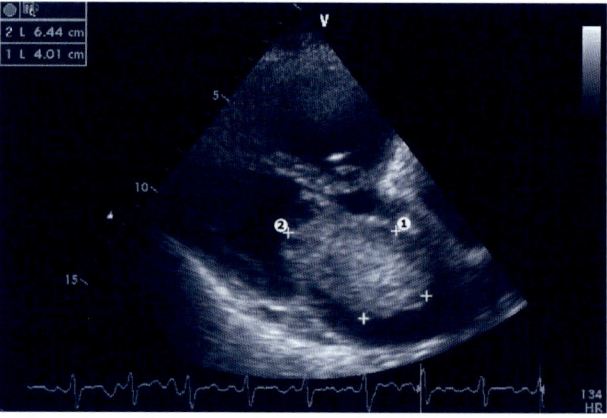

Figure 15.1 Large left atrial myxoma on transthoracic echocardiography (measurements shown).

cardiac tumours are benign, of which about 50% are myxomas. Other benign tumours of the heart include lipomas, papillary fibroelastomas and rhabdomyomas (the most common primary cardiac tumours in children). Like atria myxomas, these tumours may be asymptomatic but may also cause systemic embolism and progressive heart failure. Arrhythmias and sudden deaths have also been described with some tumours.

Primary cardiac malignancies are rare and the vast majority of these rare tumours are sarcomas. Secondary or metastatic neoplasms to the heart are far more common than primary cardiac tumours. Cardiac involvement has been described in a number of neoplasms, including lung tumours, melanoma, germ cell tumours, lymphomas, stomach, ovarian and colorectal tumours. Cardiac involvement may result in arrhythmias, progressive heart failure, pericardial effusion and tamponade. Prognosis is typically poor in patients with cardiac involvement.

How would you manage cardiac myxomas?

Surgical resection is the only effective treatment of atrial myxomas. Prior to surgery, transoesophageal echocardiography may provide additional information about the size, attachment, location and valvular involvement, all of which may guide the surgical approach. Cardiac magnetic resonance imaging may also provide useful anatomical information. Coronary angiography is generally recommended in patients with potential coronary artery disease (e.g. patients over 40 years with associated risk factors) as coronary artery bypass grafting may be performed at the time of surgery. Complete full thickness resection of the myxoma is preferred (may be difficult in the ventricle but often possible in the atrium). In this case, the atrial myxoma was completely excised and a pericardial patch used to reconstruct the atrial septum.

The prognosis of malignant cardiac sarcoma is generally poor. Haematogenous spread is common (probably due to exposure to high blood flow). Treatment of cardiac sarcomas is also limited by cardiac sensitivity to radiotherapy and potential cardiac toxicity with anthracyclines. Remission may be achieved in lymphomas.

Recurrence after surgical resection of atrial myxomas is uncommon, and may be related to incomplete resection. Recurrence in primary cardiac sarcomas is more common.

Recent Developments

Differentiation of cardiac tumours from thrombi remains a challenge in many cases. Improvements in cardiac CT and MRI have improved the diagnosis of intracardiac masses. More recently, contrast echocardiography (with intravenous injection of microbubbles which perfuse the tumour) has also been reported to be helpful in differentiating tumours from thrombi based on differences in vascularity.

Conclusion

Cardiac tumours are generally rare. Secondary or metastatic neoplasms are the most common form of cardiac tumour. Atrial myxomas are probably the most common primary cardiac tumour. Clinical presentation is varied and may be asymptomatic or include constitutional, obstructive and embolic symptoms. Transthoracic echocardiogram is a useful first-line investigation and transoesophageal echocardiogram can provide additional information to guide surgical resection. Complete full thickness resection is the only effective treatment. Recurrence rate is generally low and may be related to incomplete resection. Primary cardiac malignancies are rare and prognosis generally poor.

Further Reading

Butany J, Nair V, Naseemuddin A, Nair GM, Catton C, Yau T. Cardiac tumours: diagnosis and management. *Lancet Oncol* 2005; **6**: 219–28.

Scheffel H, Baumueller S, Stolzmann P, Leschka S, Alkadhi H, Schertler T. Atrial myxomas and thrombi: comparison of imaging features on CT. *Am J Roentgenol* 2009; **192**: 639–45.

Shapiro LM. Cardiac tumours: diagnosis and management. *Heart* 2001; **85**: 218–22.

SECTION FOUR   04

Valvular Heart Disease

16	Mitral stenosis
17	Mitral regurgitation
18	Aortic stenosis
19	Aortic regurgitation
20	Infective endocarditis

PROBLEM

16 Mitral stenosis

Case History

A 65-year-old woman presented with increasing shortness of breath on exertion over the last 3 months. She has no known cardiovascular disease but on direct questioning, revealed a history of rheumatic fever. On examination, she has a regular heart rate of 72 beats/minute and blood pressure of 138/70 mmHg. There appeared to be a loud first heart sound with a mid-diastolic murmur but examination was otherwise unremarkable.

What is the likely cause of her symptoms?

What are the causes of mitral stenosis?

What is the natural history of rheumatic mitral stenosis?

How would you investigate this patient?

Background

The clinical findings of a mid-diastolic murmur and an accentuated first heart sound are suggestive of mitral stenosis, particularly in the context of her previous history of rheumatic fever. Other clinical findings in mitral stenosis include an opening snap preceding the diastolic murmur and a pre-systolic murmur. Atrial fibrillation is a recognized association with mitral stenosis and may be the initial manifestation. Features of pulmonary hypertension (loud pulmonary second sound and parasternal heave) may also be evident.

What are the causes of mitral stenosis?

Rheumatic heart disease is the predominant cause of mitral stenosis. A history of rheumatic fever may be elicited in over 60% of patients. Other non-rheumatic causes of mitral stenosis are rare and include left atrial myxoma, mucopolysaccharidosis, severe annular calcification and autoimmune disease.

What is the natural history of rheumatic mitral stenosis?

The normal mitral valve area is about 4–5 cm^2. Symptoms are unusual with a mitral valve area of >2.5 cm^2 and resting symptoms typically occur with a valve area of <1.5 cm^2. Rheumatic mitral stenosis is a progressive and lifelong disease, with a slow stable course early on, followed by an accelerated phase later in life. A latent phase of 20–40 years from the occurrence of rheumatic fever to symptom onset is typical in developed countries. Prognosis is related to the severity of symptoms and the development of complications. The development of severe symptoms is associated with a 10-year survival of <15% and the mean survival drops to <3 years once pulmonary hypertension develops. Pulmonary or systemic congestion, systemic thromboembolism and infection are the main causes of mortality.

How would you investigate this patient?

Transthoracic echocardiography (Figure 16.1) is central to the diagnosis and assessment of mitral stenosis. Echocardiography should confirm the diagnosis and determine the severity of mitral stenosis (Table 16.1), exclude concomitant valvular abnormalities and

Table 16.1 Classification of severity of mitral stenosis

	Mild	Moderate	Severe
Mean gradient (mmHg)	<5	5–10	>10
Pulmonary arterial systolic pressure (mmHg)	<30	30–50	>50
Mitral valve area (cm^2)	>1.5	1.0–1.5	<1.0

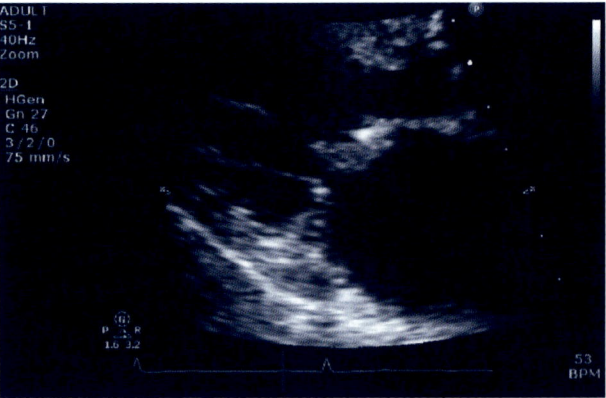

Figure 16.1 Transthoracic echocardiogram showing thickened mitral valve leaflets and restricted opening.

myocardial abnormality, estimate pulmonary artery pressure and assess the morphology of the mitral valve leaflets and subvalvular apparatus.

A scoring system – the Wilkins score – based on mitral valve and subvalvular mobility, thickening and calcification on echocardiography guides the suitability for percutaneous mitral valvotomy (Table 16.2). Percutaneous balloon valvotomy may be suitable if the Wilkins score is <8. Other contraindications to percutaneous balloon valvotomy include the presence of left atrial thrombus and concomitant moderate to severe mitral regurgitation as the procedure may worsen existing mitral regurgitation. Transoesophageal echocardiogram may also be indicated prior to percutaneous mitral valvotomy for the assessment of subvalvular fusion, commissural calcification and left atrial thrombus.

Percutaneous balloon valvotomy splits the fused commissures and a successful procedure usually doubles the mean valve area and reduces the transmitral gradient by 50–60%. Clinical studies suggest 80–90% event-free survival over 307 years of follow-up with percutaneous balloon valvotomy if valvular anatomy is suitable, which compares favourably with surgical commissurotomy or valve replacement. In experienced centres, the procedure has a low complication rate (mitral regurgitation, atrial septal defect, ventricular perforation and death) of <3%. Therefore, percutaneous balloon valvotomy should be considered the initial treatment of choice in symptomatic patients with severe mitral stenosis with favourable valvular anatomy (Figure 16.2).

Finally, the patient's heart rhythm should be documented, as atrial fibrillation is frequently associated with mitral stenosis because of left atrial dilatation. The development of atrial fibrillation results in the loss of atrial contribution to ventricular filling and clinical deterioration. Initial treatment of atrial fibrillation should include anticoagulation and rate control with digoxin, β-blocker or calcium channel antagonist. Emergency cardioversion should be considered in cases of haemodynamic instability. In this case, the patient is in sinus rhythm. Atrial fibrillation in a patient with mitral stenosis is associated with significant risk of thromboembolism and anticoagulation is strongly recommended in these patients.

Table 16.2 Wilkins classification

Grade	Mobility	Subvalvular thickening	Valvular thickening	Calcification
1	High mobile valve with only leaflet tips restricted	Minimal thickening just below the mitral leaflets	Leaflets nearly normal in thickness (4–5 mm)	Single area of increased echo brightness
2	Leaflet mid- and basal portions normally mobile	Thickening of chordal structures extending up to one-third of chordal length	Mid leaflets normal, considerable thickening of margins (5–8 mm)	Scattered areas of brightness confined to leaflet margins
3	Valve continues to move forward in diastole, mainly from base	Thickening extending to the distal third of chords	Thickening extending through the entire leaflet (5–8 mm)	Brightness extending into mid-portion of leaflets
4	No or minimal forward movement of the leaflets in diastole	Extensive thickening and shortening of all chordal structures extending down to papillary muscles	Considerable thickening of all leaflet tissue (>8–10 mm)	Extensive brightness throughout much of of the leaflet tissue

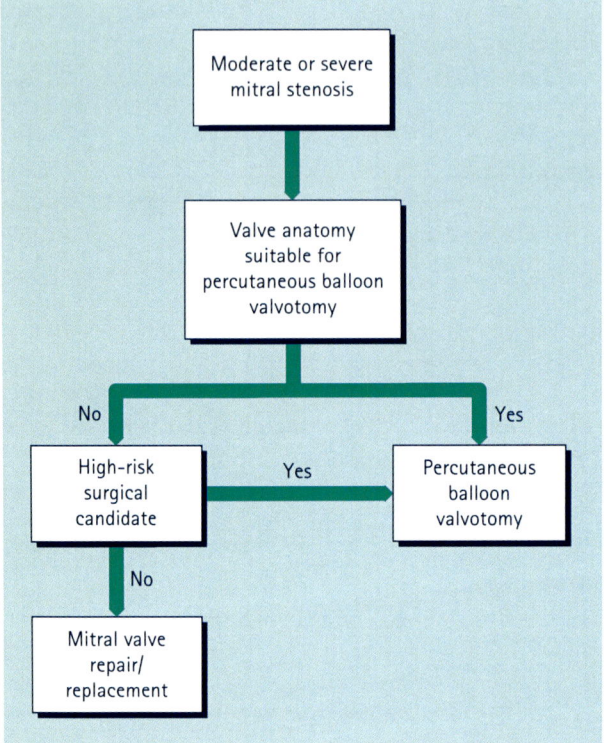

Figure 16.2 Management of mitral stenosis.

Recent Developments

 Echocardiography has conventionally been used to assess the severity of mitral stenosis. Recently, multislice computed tomography has been used to assess mitral valve area in mitral stenosis and shown to correlate well with echocardiographic measurements.

Conclusion

 Rheumatic heart disease is the most common cause of mitral stenosis. Percutaneous balloon valvotomy should be considered the initial treatment of choice in patients with symptomatic mitral stenosis, particularly if the anatomy of the mitral valve and subvalvular apparatus is favourable. The development of atrial fibrillation may result in clinical deterioration and carries a high risk of thromboembolism. Anticoagulation and rate control should be instituted early and emergency cardioversion if there is evidence of haemodynamic instability.

Further Reading

Bonow RO, Carabello BA, Chatterjee K, et al. ACC/AHA 2006 guidelines for the management of patients with valvular heart disease: a report of the American College of Cardiology/American Heart Association Task Force on Practice Guidelines. *J Am Coll Cardiol* 2006; **48**: e1–148.

Zoghbi WA, Enriquez-Sarano M, Foster E, et al. Recommendations for evaluation of the severity of native valvular regurgitation with two-dimensional and Doppler echocardiography. *J Am Soc Echocardiogr* 2003; **16**: 777–802.

PROBLEM

17 Mitral regurgitation

Case History

A 65-year-old woman complained of increasing shortness of breath on exertion over the last 6 months with significant deterioration over the last 2 weeks. She denied any exertional chest pain or nocturnal breathlessness. She has a history of hypertension, which appears to be adequately controlled by perindopril. She recalled a previous diagnosis of a murmur over 10 years ago and investigations, then suggested minor leaking of one of her heart valves. She failed to attend further appointments following the investigations. On examination, her pulse was irregular at 120 beats/minute with a blood pressure of 122/78 mmHg. There was a clear pan-systolic murmur throughout the precordium but her heart sounds were otherwise normal. Her apex beat was displaced towards the axilla. Clinical examination was otherwise unremarkable.

What do the clinical findings suggest?

How would you manage this patient?

Background

Clinical assessment of a patient with chronic mitral regurgitation should establish baseline exercise tolerance and the degree of symptomatic limitation. Physical examination typically reveals a pan-systolic murmur, which may radiate into the axilla, which may be associated with a third heart sound. Atrial fibrillation (irregular pulse) and features of heart failure should be sought and a displaced apex beat may suggest left ventricular enlargement. Clinical features of pulmonary hypertension would suggest significant chronic mitral regurgitation. The clinical findings in this patient are therefore consistent with mitral regurgitation associated with left ventricular dilatation and atrial fibrillation.

How would you manage this patient?

Clinical findings should be correlated with those from transthoracic echocardiography, which is central for baseline assessment of the severity of mitral regurgitation (Table 17.1), possible mechanism for mitral regurgitation (e.g. mitral valve prolapse, rheumatic heart disease or secondary to annular dilatation), left ventricular size and systolic function, left atrial size and estimated pulmonary artery pressure. Assessment of left ventricular function by ejection fraction is difficult as regurgitation into the low pressure left atrium increases the measured ejection fraction and may mask deterioration in systolic function. Therefore, a higher cut-off of at least 60% is used to define normal left ventricular systolic function in the presence of mitral regurgitation. A central jet of mitral regurgitation with a structurally normal mitral valve usually indicates functional mitral regurgitation (secondary to mitral annular dilatation). Calcification of the valvular apparatus, redundancy of the valve leaflets (e.g. in mitral valve prolapse) and the leaflets involved may guide the type of mitral valve surgery.

Transoesophageal echocardiography is indicated for further characterization of the anatomy of the mitral valve prior to surgery and in cases when transthoracic echocardiographic assessments are inconclusive. Left ventriculography, haemodynamic measurements of pulmonary artery pressure and coronary angiography are indicated if data from non-invasive testing are inconclusive and in patients at risk of coronary artery disease. In this case, transthoracic echocardiography demonstrated prolapse of the posterior mitral valve leaflet (defined as prolapse of >2 mm above the mitral annulus) with redundant and thickened mitral valve leaflets, left ventricular dilatation but ejection fraction of 50%, but no evidence of pulmonary hypertension (Figure 17.1 – see inside front cover for part (a)). Coronary angiography did not show any obstructive coronary artery disease. Of note, the classic mid-systolic clicks may be absent in patients with typical echocardiographic features of mitral valve prolapse.

Table 17.1 Assessment of the severity of mitral regurgitation

	Mild	Moderate	Severe
Qualitative			
Angiographic grade	1+	2+↓	3–4+↓
Colour Doppler jet area*	<20% LA area	20–40%	>40% LA area
Vena contracta (cm)	>0.3	0.3–0.69	≥0.7
Quantitative+			
Regurgitant volume (ml/beat)	<30		>60
Regurgitant fraction (%)	<30	30–49	>50
Regurgitant orifice area (cm²)	<0.2	0.2–0.39	≥0.4

*May be underestimated in eccentric mitral regurgitation jets.
**Quantitative assessment by either ventriculography or echocardiography.

17 Mitral regurgitation

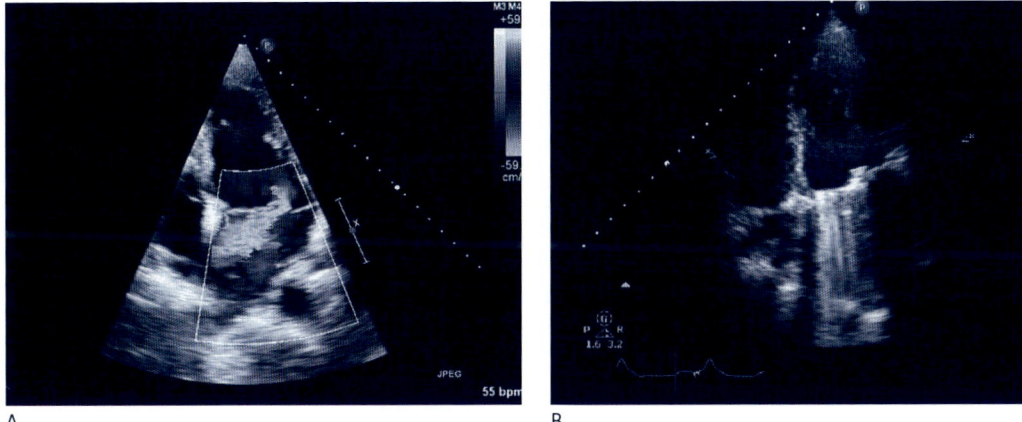

Figure 17.1 (A) Severe mitral regurgitation on colour Doppler echocardiography. (B) Prosthetic mitral valve with acoustic shadow on echocardiogram (see inside front cover for colour version).

Patients with severe mitral regurgitation who are apparently asymptomatic should undergo exercise testing for objective assessment of exercise tolerance. The exercise test may be combined with transthoracic echocardiography to assess the effects of exercise on the severity of mitral regurgitation and pulmonary artery pressure.

Unfortunately, there is no established medical treatment for patients with chronic mitral regurgitation. Although vasodilators are used in patients with acute severe mitral regurgitation, they have no established benefit in patients with isolated chronic mitral regurgitation. Angiotensin-converting enzyme inhibitors may be used for concomitant arterial hypertension or left ventricular dysfunction, but they have not been shown to alter the progression of mitral regurgitation. This patient was commenced on a β-blocker for ventricular rate control and warfarin for the prevention of thromboembolism associated with atrial fibrillation. She was aware of the need for antibiotic prophylaxis against infective endocarditis.

The indications for mitral valve surgery are listed in Table 17.2. Mitral valve surgery has evolved significantly with growing appreciation for the role of the mitral valve apparatus in maintaining left ventricular geometry and function. There are now three types of surgical operations for mitral regurgitation: (1) mitral valve repair; (2) mitral valve replacement with preservation of either part or all of the mitral valve apparatus; and (3) mitral valve replacement with resection of the mitral valve apparatus. Preservation of the mitral valve apparatus preserves left ventricular shape and function, and is associated with better postoperative cardiac function. Indeed, mitral valve repair should be considered the operation of choice (particularly in mitral valve prolapse) if the valvular

---

Table 17.2 Class I indications for surgery

- Symptomatic acute severe mitral regurgitation.
- Symptomatic chronic severe mitral regurgitation in the absence of severe left ventricle dysfunction (ejection fraction <30% and/or end-systolic diameter of >55 mm).
- Asymptomatic patients with chronic severe mitral regurgitation and mild-to-moderate left ventricle dysfunction (ejection fraction 30–60% and/or end-systolic diameter 40 mm or more).

anatomy is suitable as it not only preserves the valvular apparatus but also spares the patient from long-term anticoagulation. However, mitral valve repair is technically more demanding although the reoperation rate is similar to mitral valve replacement surgery (7–10% at 10 years) in experienced centres. Repair of the posterior compared with the anterior mitral valve leaflet is associated with a lower reoperation rate. Mitral valve replacement with resection of valve apparatus is rarely performed and is usually reserved for patients with a severely distorted valvular anatomy (e.g. severe calcification).

Management of a patient with severe symptomatic mitral regurgitation associated with severe left ventricular dysfunction (ejection fraction <30%) is difficult (Figure 17.2). Clinical outcome from mitral valve surgery in these patients is compromised by the poor left ventricular function and the decision to proceed with surgery will need to be individualized.

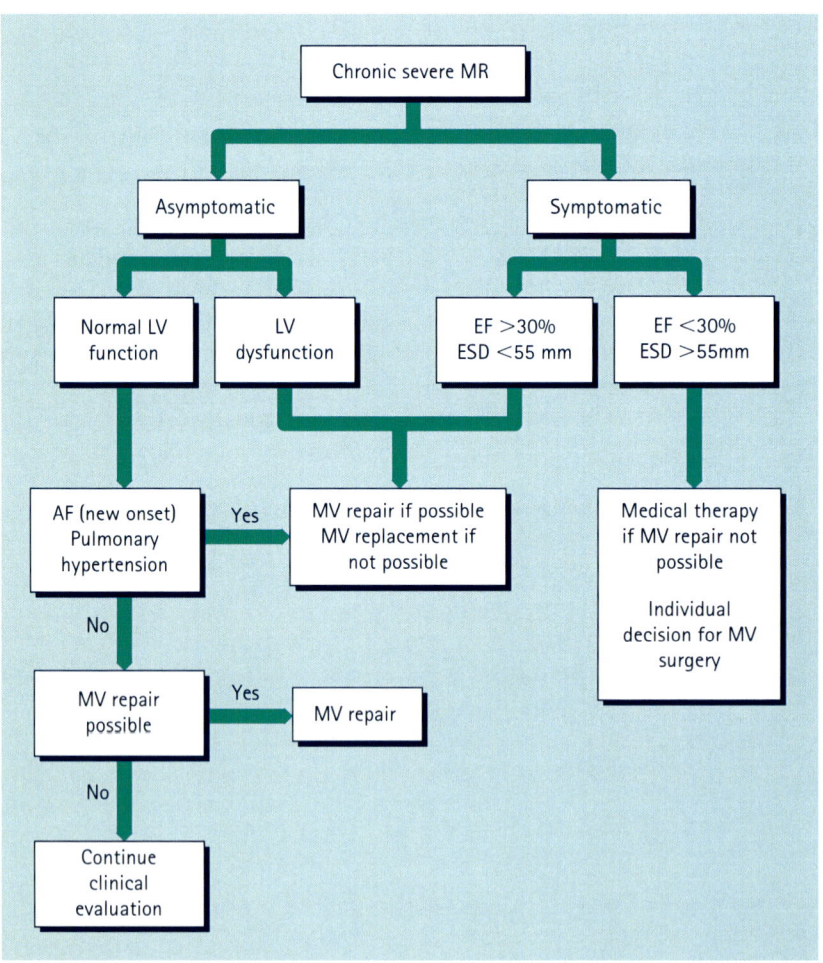

Figure 17.2 Management of mitral regurgitation. AF, atrial fibrillation; EF, ejection fraction; ESD, end-systolic dimension; LV, left ventricular; MR, mitral regurgitation.

Mitral regurgitation is frequently associated with atrial fibrillation because of the haemodynamic load on the left atrium. The development of atrial fibrillation may be associated with clinical deterioration and may be regarded as an indication for mitral valve surgery in patients with severe mitral regurgitation. A concomitant ablation procedure (Maze procedure) may restore sinus rhythm and may be considered with mitral valve surgery if technically feasible. In this case, the patient's mitral valve anatomy was suitable for repair and she underwent successful mitral valve repair surgery with atrial fibrillation ablation surgery.

This case relates to a patient with primary organic mitral regurgitation, which is pathophysiologically distinct from mitral regurgitation secondary to annular dilatation (left ventricular dilatation) and ischaemia. The latter may be a consequence of local ventricular remodelling, which results in displacement of the papillary muscle and tethering of the mitral valve. The mitral valve itself is usually structurally normal. Mitral valve repair at the time of surgical revascularization (coronary bypass grafting surgery) may improve mitral regurgitation over revascularization alone. Therefore, patients with ischaemic heart disease should be assessed for mitral regurgitation prior to coronary surgery.

Recent Developments

Mitral regurgitation in the context of ischaemic heart disease is associated with poorer outcomes. Ischaemic mitral regurgitation is not usually due to intrinsic valvular abnormality but, rather, reflects abnormalities in the ventricle, such as displacement of the posterior papillary muscle, ventricular enlargement with increased ventricular sphericity, which displaces both papillary muscles, annular enlargement, papillary muscle dyssynchrony, and reduced leaflet-closing force from left ventricular dysfunction. The best method of reducing ischaemic mitral regurgitation, however, is not clear. Mitral valve replacement is associated with the possibility of further deterioration in left ventricle function and complications associated with prosthetic valves. Restrictive mitral annuloplasty (insertion of an undersized annular ring to improve apposition of the mitral valve) has been used for over a decade, but recent data have reported a recurrence of mitral regurgitation in a significant proportion of patients and even functional mitral stenosis with this technique. Recurrence of mitral regurgitation is likely to be due to progressive remodelling of the left ventricle. Hence, ongoing studies will evaluate novel surgical techniques to overcome the alteration in left ventricle shape that drive ischaemic mitral regurgitation.

Developments in imaging technology, in particular real-time three-dimensional transthoracic and transoesophageal echocardiography, have improved visualization of mitral valve anatomy and complement advances in surgical repair techniques. Real-time three-dimensional transthoracic echocardiography may even be superior to conventional two-dimensional transoesophageal echocardiography.

Conclusion

Untreated severe mitral regurgitation results in progressive pump failure, arrhythmias, pulmonary hypertension and death. Early correction of severe mitral regurgitation before left ventricular dysfunction develops is associated with better clinical outcomes. Careful evaluation (clinical, invasive and non-invasive assessment) may identify patients who will benefit from surgery and guide surgical treatment. Assessment of left ventricular function should take into consideration the effect of mitral regurgitation and a higher threshold of 60% ejection fraction should be regarded as normal in these patients. Finally, mitral valve repair is preferable if the anatomy is suitable.

Further Reading

Bonow RO, Carabello BA, Chatterjee K, *et al.* ACC/AHA 2006 guidelines for the management of patients with valvular heart disease: a report of the American College of Cardiology/American Heart Association Task Force on Practice Guidelines. *J Am Coll Cardiol* 2006; **48**: e1–148.

Enriquez-Sarano M, Tribouilloy C. Quantification of mitral regurgitation: rationale, approach and interpretation in clinical practice. *Heart* 2002; **88**(Suppl. 4): 1–3.

PROBLEM

18 Aortic stenosis

Case History

An 80-year-old man presented with a 6-month history of gradually increasing breathlessness on exertion. He has no known heart disease and is a non-smoker. He has a history of hypertension, which is controlled on a thiazide diuretic. He has no history of rheumatic fever. On examination, his pulse was regular and blood pressure was measured at 130/70 mmHg. His chest was clear but he had a clear ejection systolic murmur that radiated to his carotid arteries. His venous pressure was not elevated and he had no peripheral oedema. His ECG is as shown in Figure 18.1. The ECG confirmed sinus rhythm and fulfilled the voltage criteria for left ventricular hypertrophy.

What would be your initial differential diagnosis?

How would you investigate this patient?

How would you manage this patient?

Would you manage this patient differently if he had poor left ventricular function?

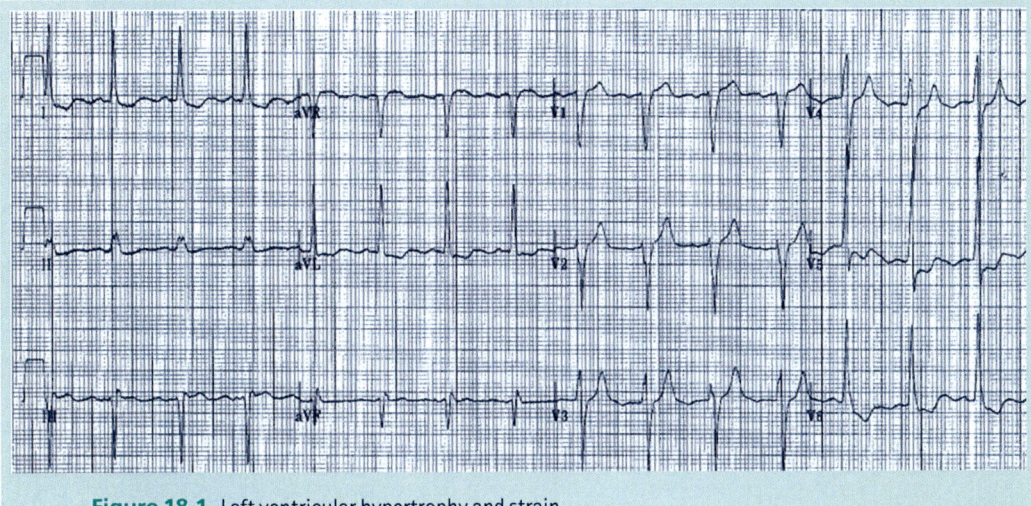

Figure 18.1 Left ventricular hypertrophy and strain.

Background

 Left ventricular hypertrophy (LVH) is often a result of uncontrolled high blood pressure. However, obstruction of the left ventricular outflow tract, and aortic stenosis in particular, is also a major cause of LVH. This must be considered the primary differential diagnosis in the context of an elderly man with ejection systolic murmur typical of aortic stenosis and controlled blood pressure. Hypertrophic cardiomyopathy is another cause of LVH.

How would you investigate this patient?

Transthoracic echocardiography is recommended for the diagnosis and assessment of the severity of aortic stenosis. The latter may be defined by a number of measurements obtained by echocardiography, including valve morphology (and the degree of calcification) and opening, peak and mean pressure gradient estimated by Doppler echocardiography across the aortic valve and the estimated aortic valve area (Table 18.1). Left

Table 18.1 Severity of aortic stenosis

Severity	Echocardiographic measurements
Mild	Mean gradient <25 mmHg Valve area >1.5 cm²
Moderate	Mean gradient 25–40 mmHg Valve area 1.0–1.5 cm²
Severe	Mean gradient >40 mmHg Valve area <1.0 cm²

ventricular size and function may also be measured from echocardiography. The assessment of other concomitant valvular abnormalities is also crucial, particularly if there is a history of rheumatic fever, as involvement of the mitral valve is almost invariable in the presence of rheumatic aortic stenosis.

Exercise testing may be considered in the asymptomatic individual with aortic stenosis to assess functional capacity, symptoms and blood pressure response. Owing to stenosis of the aortic outflow, vasodilatation during exercise may not be matched by an increase in cardiac output, which may result in a drop in blood pressure and haemodynamic compromise. Therefore, blood pressure drop in a patient with aortic valve disease during exercise suggests significant stenosis. Exercise testing should be performed only under medical supervision and should not be performed in symptomatic patients.

In this case, echocardiogram confirms severe aortic stenosis with LVH but normal systolic function (ejection fraction >50%) (Figure 18.2).

How would you manage this patient?

There is no proven medical treatment for aortic stenosis (Figure 18.3). Lipid-lowering therapy with statins has been tried previously to delay the progression of aortic valve dis-

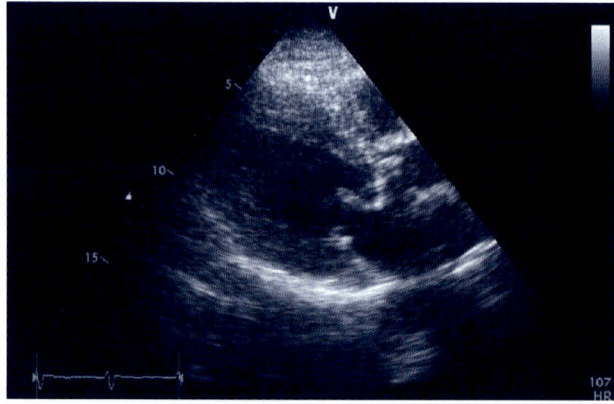

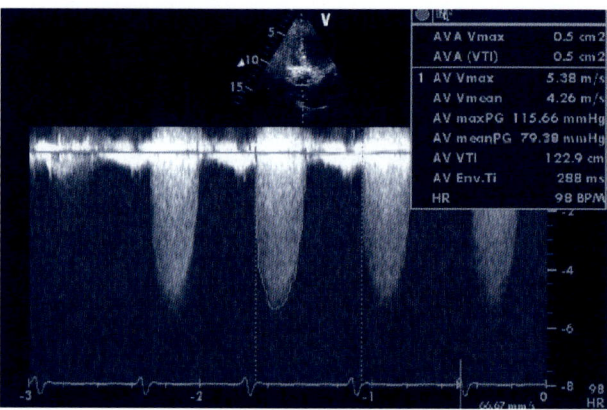

Figure 18.2 (A) Thickened aortic valve on transthoracic echocardiogram. (B) High gradient across aortic valve on Doppler echocardiogram.

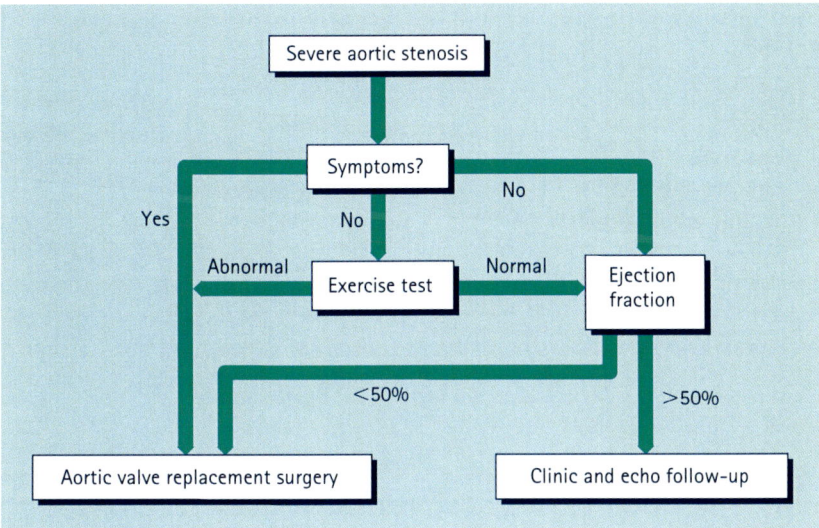

Figure 18.3 Management of aortic stenosis.

ease on the basis of overlapping pathophysiology with atherosclerotic coronary artery disease, but this was not supported by randomized studies to date. Aortic valve replacement (AVR) is indicated in patients with symptomatic severe aortic stenosis in the absence of other significant comorbidities. Age alone is not a contraindication to surgery as many of these patients can expect a favourable outcome from surgery. The patient in this case should therefore be considered for AVR. The role for percutaneous aortic valvuloplasty is limited although percutaneous AVR is currently under development.

In preparation for AVR, coronary angiography is indicated to assess the coronary circulation and the need for coronary bypass grafting surgery at the time of AVR surgery. In some cases, a right heart catheterization may also be performed to assess the haemodynamic effects of aortic valve disease particularly if data from transthoracic echocardiography are not conclusive. Cardiac catheterization for haemodynamic measurements and assessment of aortic stenosis should not be routinely performed if data from non-invasive tests are adequate.

The management of the asymptomatic patient with severe aortic stenosis, however, is more controversial. Early AVR will expose these asymptomatic patients to the risks of morbidity and mortality associated with prosthetic valves and in the case of bioprosthetic valves, structural deterioration of the bioprosthesis and need for earlier replacement. Some would advocate early AVR even in the absence of symptoms on the basis that 50% of patients will develop symptoms in 5 years and to prevent potentially irreversible myocardial damage from untreated, persistently elevated afterload, although the latter has yet to be proven. Others suggest closer monitoring of clinical and echocardiographic parameters to identify patients whose aortic valve disease may progress rapidly. In general, patients over 50 years of age with significant valvular calcification and concomitant coronary artery disease are likely to progress more rapidly.

Would you manage this patient differently if he had poor left ventricular function?

Patients with severe aortic stenosis and depressed left ventricular function often present with only low-pressure gradient and may be difficult to distinguish from patients with low-pressure gradient due primarily to contractile dysfunction. In the latter, the low ejection fraction and failure to generate adequate stroke volume result in limited valve opening and apparent aortic stenosis (pseudo-aortic stenosis). The distinction between these two entities is crucial as AVR may alleviate the significant afterload associated with severe aortic stenosis, which may result in some recovery of left ventricular function in true aortic stenosis, but will have no value in patients with pseudo-aortic stenosis. Dobutamine stress echocardiography to increase stroke volume may help in the diagnosis.

Recent Developments

The technique of percutaneous aortic valve implantation has undergone considerable advances over the last few years. The feasibility of this technique is now established. Percutaneous aortic valve implantation has also been shown to provide haemodynamic and clinical improvement for up to 2 years in patients with severe symptomatic aortic stenosis at high risk or with contraindications for surgery. Future studies will assess the long-term durability and clinical outcomes of this technique.

Conclusion

Transthoracic echocardiography is central to the diagnosis and assessment of a patient with aortic stenosis. Additional non-invasive testing may be needed, particularly in the asymptomatic patient. Patients with symptomatic severe aortic stenosis should be considered for AVR surgery in view of the extremely poor prognosis if left untreated.

Further Reading

Bonow RO, Carabello BA, Chatterjee K, *et al.* ACC/AHA 2006 guidelines for the management of patients with valvular heart disease: a report of the American College of Cardiology/American Heart Association Task Force on Practice Guidelines. *J Am Coll Cardiol* 2006; **48**: e1–148.

Vahanian A, Alfieri O, Al-Attar N, *et al.* Transcatheter valve implantation for patients with aortic stenosis: a position statement from the European Association of Cardio-Thoracic Surgery (EACTS) and the European Society of Cardiology (ESC), in collaboration with the European Association of Percutaneous Cardiovascular Interventions (EAPCI). *Eur Heart J* 2008; **29**: 1463–70.

19 Aortic regurgitation

Case History

A 72-year-old man presented with exertional central chest tightness and shortness of breath over the last 3 months. He has a long history of hypertension treated with a thiazide diuretic. He also takes a statin regularly for primary prevention and has no known cardiac disease. He is an ex-smoker. On examination, his blood pressure was 180/72 mmHg and he was in sinus rhythm. There was a systolic murmur, an audible early diastolic murmur and a third heart sound. His venous pressure was not elevated and he had no peripheral oedema.

What do you think is the cause of his symptoms?

How would you investigate this man?

How would you treat this man?

What if this patient has asymptomatic severe aortic regurgitation?

Background

This man's exertional symptoms are suggestive of coronary artery disease, particularly in view of his age and long-standing hypertension. However, his wide pulse pressure, diastolic murmur and third heart sound should raise the suspicion of aortic regurgitation. Exertional chest pain is not uncommon in patients with aortic regurgitation and may in part be related to a reduced coronary flow reserve as a consequence of left ventricular hypertrophy.

How would you investigate this man?

Transthoracic echocardiography is recommended for the diagnosis and the assessment of the severity of aortic regurgitation. The latter may be defined by a number of measurements obtained by echocardiography, including valve morphology (and the degree of calcification) and semi-quantitative and quantitative measurements of the severity of aortic regurgitation (Table 19.1) and aortic root dimensions. Left ventricular size and function should also be measured, as increased left ventricular dimensions and reduced function are associated with worse prognosis and higher operative risks. Radionuclide ventriculography or cardiac magnetic resonance imaging (MRI) may be indicated for the assessment of left ventricular volumes if echocardiographic assessment is inadequate. Exercise testing may be considered in the asymptomatic individual with aortic regurgitation to assess functional capacity and symptoms in response to exercise. In this case, transthoracic

Table 19.1 Severity of aortic regurgitation			
	Mild	Moderate	Severe
Colour Doppler jet width	<25% of LVOT	25–65% of LVOT	>65% of LVOT
Doppler vena contracta	<0.3 cm	0.3–0.6 cm	>0.6 cm
Regurgitant volume (ml/beat)	<30	30–59	≥60
Regurgitant fraction (%)	<30	30–49	≥50
Regurgitant orifice area (cm^2)	<0.10	0.10–0.29	≥0.3

LVOT, left ventricular outflow tract.

echocardiogram confirms severe aortic regurgitation with a dilated left ventricle with normal ejection fraction (>50%). Other coexistent valvular abnormalities should be assessed by transthoracic or transoesophageal echocardiography (Figure 19.1 demonstrates aortic regurgitation on transoesophageal echocardiogram [see inside front cover]).

How would you treat this man?

Vasodilators have been used for the treatment of aortic regurgitation on the basis that they increase forward flow and reduce regurgitant volume. A recent study of 95 patients with aortic regurgitation compared long-acting nifedipine, enalapril and placebo, and found no significant difference in the development of symptoms or left ventricular dysfunction warranting aortic valve surgery over 7 years. Hence, there is no definitive recommendation for long-term vasodilator treatment for the asymptomatic patient with severe aortic regurgitation. Vasodilators, however, may be used for the treatment of systolic hypertension frequently observed in these patients due to the increased stroke volume. It is rarely possible to 'normalize' systolic blood pressure and, indeed, vasodilators should not be used in excessive doses in an attempt to achieve normal systolic blood pressure. Specifically, vasodilators are not indicated in patients with mild–moderate aortic regurgitation and are not a substitute for aortic valve surgery in patients with severe aortic regurgitation, although they may be used to optimize heart failure therapy in the short term in preparation for surgery.

Aortic valve replacement surgery is indicated in this case of symptomatic severe aortic regurgitation. In preparation for aortic valve replacement, coronary angiography is indicated to assess the coronary circulation and the need for coronary bypass grafting surgery at the time of aortic valve replacement surgery. In addition, a root aortogram should be performed during angiography to assess aortic root dimension (and the need for aortic root surgery) unless this is adequately demonstrated by other non-invasive imaging (e.g. computed tomography or MRI of the aorta). Right heart catheterization is not routinely performed for the assessment of the haemodynamic effects of aortic valve disease.

What if this patient has asymptomatic, severe aortic regurgitation?

Long-term results of aortic valve surgery are now generally favourable, with mortality more closely related to pre-operative myocardial function than the surgery itself. Nonetheless, aortic valve replacement surgery in an asymptomatic patient with severe

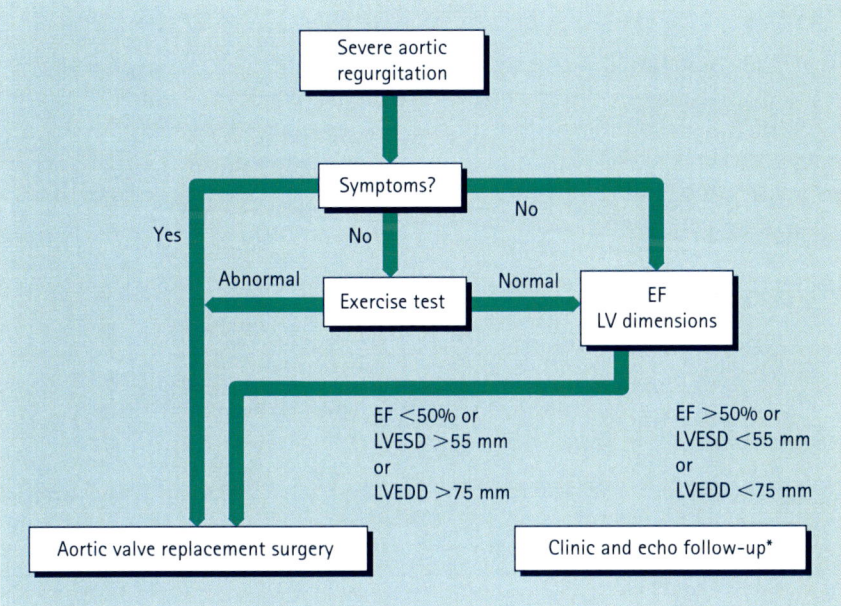

Figure 19.2 Management of severe aortic regurgitation. [*]Frequency of follow-up is dependent on the LV dimensions and stability of these measurements over time. EF, ejection fraction; LV, left ventricular; LVEDD, left ventricular end-diastolic diameter; LVESD, left ventricular end-systolic diameter.

aortic regurgitation is controversial. Current guidelines recommend the measurement of left ventricular dimensions and function to guide the timing for aortic valve surgery (Figure 19.2). Based on a number of small longitudinal studies, aortic valve surgery is recommended if severe aortic regurgitation is associated with depressed systolic function (ejection fraction <50%) or left ventricular dilatation (end-systolic diameter >55 mm and end-systolic diameter >75 mm). In order to overcome the inherent variability in the measurement of ejection fraction or left ventricular dimensions, more than one measurement is recommended. The second measurement may be obtained through a different imaging modality such as cardiac MRI.

Recent Developments

Bicuspid aortic valve is one of the most common causes of aortic regurgitation, particularly in those under the age of 65 years. Replacement of the aortic valve, whether mechanical or bioprosthetic is limited by the need for long-term anticoagulation (and associated bleeding risks) and late failure of the bioprosthesis. There is now growing interest in identifying valves suitable for repair based on detailed characterization of valvular anatomy (e.g. thickening or calcification of commissures and cusps and valve coaptation) and valve tissue 'quality'. The feasibility and long-term outcome of aortic valve repair needs further study.

Conclusion

Exertional chest pain is a recognized presentation for aortic regurgitation. Vasodilators have only a limited role in the management of severe aortic regurgitation. Aortic valve replacement is recommended for symptomatic aortic regurgitation. Assessment of the aortic root dimensions should be routine prior to aortic valve surgery in view of the recognized association between aortic root dilatation and aortic regurgitation.

Further Reading

Bonow RO, Carabello BA, Chatterjee K, *et al.* ACC/AHA 2006 guidelines for the management of patients with valvular heart disease: a report of the American College of Cardiology/American Heart Association Task Force on Practice Guidelines. *J Am Coll Cardiol* 2006; **48**: e1–148.

Sambola A, Tornos P, Ferreira-Gonzalez I, Evangelista A. Prognostic value of preoperative indexed end-systolic left ventricle diameter in the outcome after surgery in patients with chronic aortic regurgitation. *Am Heart J* 2008; **155**: 1114–20.

PROBLEM

20 Infective endocarditis

Case History

An 80-year-old man underwent an uncomplicated (bioprosthetic) aortic valve replacement for calcific aortic stenosis. He has a history of hypertension but no significant coronary artery disease. On the eighth postoperative day, he developed a pyrexial episode of 39°C. He felt generally unwell but no specific symptoms. Clinical examination did not reveal any splinter haemorrhages or any signs of embolic complications. The sternal wound looked well healed. There was a soft diastolic murmur and an ejection systolic murmur but no evidence of heart failure.

What do you think is the cause of this man's pyrexial illness?

How would you manage this case?

20 Infective endocarditis

Background

Postoperative pyrexial illness is typically related to infective complications. In a patient who has recently undergone valve replacement surgery, infective endocarditis of the prosthetic valve must be considered. Some cases may also be complicated by infective mediastinitis. Other postoperative complications include pneumonia, infected intravenous lines and urinary catheters. In this case, a chest radiograph did not demonstrate any evidence of a pneumonic complication. Urinary dipstick demonstrated haematuria but urine culture did not yield any significant growth. Three sets of blood cultures were taken and staphylococcus was grown in all three sets after 3 days. This was later identified as *Staphylococcus epidermidis*. There was no external evidence of infection to explain the staphylococcal bacteraemia. He was commenced on antibiotics even before the results of the blood cultures were available. Staphylococcal endocarditis was therefore the most likely diagnosis.

How would you manage this case?

Transthoracic echocardiography is generally recommended to detect valvular vegetations/abscess and the severity of valvular dysfunction (Figure 20.1). However, the sensitivity of transthoracic echocardiography for detecting valvular vegetations is limited. Three echocardiographic findings are considered major criteria in the diagnosis of infective endocarditis:

- A mobile, echodense mass attached to the valvular/mural endocardium or to implanted prosthetic material.
- Demonstration of abscesses or fistulas.
- A new dehiscence of valve prosthesis, especially late after implantation.

A transthoracic echocardiogram was performed in this case with acquisition of good images. The transthoracic echocardiogram did not show obvious vegetations, but there was moderate transvalvular aortic regurgitation across the aortic valve prosthesis. There

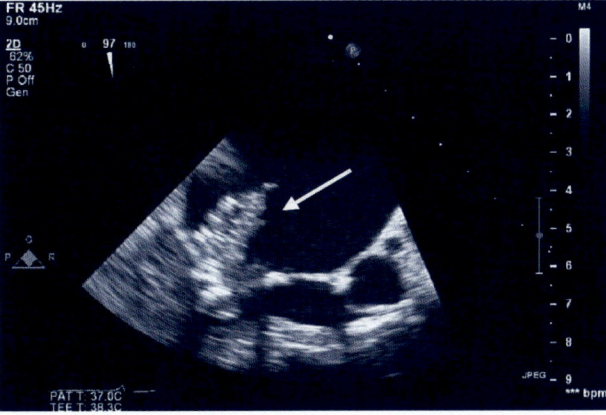

Figure 20.1 Large vegetation on mitral valve (arrow) demonstrated on transoesophageal echocardiography.

was no evidence of valve dehiscence or abscess. Electrocardiogram did not show any evidence of atrioventricular conduction delay, which may be a complication of bacterial endocarditis (infiltrating the conduction tissue).

The variable presentation of infective endocarditis often presents considerable diagnostic difficulties. The Duke criteria initially proposed over a decade ago have undergone modifications to take into consideration the greater use of transoesophageal echocardiography, increasing prevalence of staphylococcal infection and recognition of Q fever endocarditis (*Coxiella burnetti*). Clinical studies suggest that these modifications improve the diagnosis of infective endocarditis. The modified Duke criteria are listed in Table 20.1. Based on the investigations outlined above, this case fulfils the pathological criteria, two major (new valvular regurgitation and positive blood cultures) and two minor (pyrexia and predisposing heart condition) criteria. Thus, based on the modified Duke criteria, this man has 'definite' infective endocarditis.

It is clear from the diagnostic criteria that blood cultures are crucial to the diagnosis of bacterial endocarditis. At least 10 ml of blood should be taken following antiseptic skin preparation to avoid contamination. Most guidelines recommend at least three sets of blood cultures as in this case. As bacteraemia is continuous, the collection of blood cul-

Table 20.1 Modified Duke diagnostic criteria

Pathological criteria
Microorganism demonstrated by culture/histological examination
Active endocarditis on histological examination

Major criteria
Positive blood cultures
- Typical organism consistent with endocarditis on two separate blood cultures (streptococci, HACEK group, *Staphylococcus aureus*, enterococci)
- Organism consistent with endocarditis from persistently positive blood cultures
- Positive serology for *Coxiella burnetti*, *Chlamydia psitacci* and *Bartonella* species

Evidence of endocardial involvement
Echocardiographic evidence (e.g. oscillating structure, abscess, dehiscence of prosthetic valve)
New valvular regurgitation

Minor criteria
Predisposing heart condition (e.g. prosthetic heart valve) or *intravenous drug use*

Fever >38°C

Vascular phenomenon (embolic complications, mycotic aneurysm, intracranial haemorrhage, conjunctival haemorrhage, Janeway's lesions)

Immunological phenomenon (rheumatoid factor, glomerulonephritis, Osler's nodes, Roth spots)

Microbiological evidence not meeting major criteria

Echocardiographic changes not meeting major criteria

DEFINITE ENDOCARDITIS
Pathological criteria plus 2 major, or 1 major and 3 minor, or 5 minor criteria

POSSIBLE ENDOCARDITIS
1 major and 1 minor, or 3 minor criteria

REJECTED
Firm alternative diagnosis
Resolution after <4 days of antibiotic therapy
Does not meet criteria above
HACEK bacteria (*h*aemophilus, *a*ctinobacillus, *c*ardiobacterium, *e*ikenella, *k*ingella)

tures does not need to coincide with pyrexial episodes. Blood cultures may be negative in up to 30% of cases and may be due to previous antibiotic treatment or fastidious organisms, which may require an alternative culture medium or diagnostic technique (e.g. serology). Causes of apparently negative blood cultures are listed in Table 20.2.

Transoesophageal echocardiography has a role in the diagnosis of infective endocarditis, particularly if transthoracic echocardiography is non-diagnostic and the associated complications (e.g. perivalvular abscess) are suspected (Figure 20.1). In cases of suspected prosthetic valve endocarditis, transoesophageal echocardiography has even been recommended as the first-line diagnostic study. Some clinical studies suggest that valvular vegetations may be detectable by transoesophageal echocardiography in over 90% of cases.

Bactericidal antibiotics are central to the effective treatment of bacterial endocarditis. High serum antibiotic concentrations are generally desirable to ensure adequate penetration into vegetations, which are typically enclosed in polysaccharides hampering antibiotic penetration. Intravenous antibiotics are preferred to ensure maximal bioavailability. The choice and duration of antibiotic therapy depend on the organism, again emphasizing the importance of identifying the organism. The majority of cases (80%) of infective endocarditis are caused by streptococci or staphylococci. Early prosthetic valve endocarditis (conventionally defined as <2 months) is usually caused by *Staphylococcus epidermidis* as in this case.

Benzylpenicillin plus gentamicin is generally recommended for streptococcal endocarditis. Vancomycin may be used in patients intolerant of penicillin. In cases of uncomplicated native valve endocarditis, 2–4 weeks of treatment may be adequate. Infections due to *Staphylococcus aureus* require a longer duration (6 weeks) of treatment usually consisting of flucloxacillin (or vancomycin) plus gentamicin. Similarly, enterococcal endocarditis requires up to 6 weeks of treatment.

Staphylococcal infection of prosthetic valves is treated more aggressively and a combination of gentamicin, vancomycin and rifampicin is recommended, usually for at least 6 weeks. In this case, the patient was treated with a combination of gentamicin, vancomycin and rifampicin. However, the patient continued to deteriorate clinically with the development of symptoms and signs of heart failure. A transoesophageal echocardiogram was performed for further assessment of valvular dysfunction and complications.

Table 20.2 **Causes of culture-negative infective endocarditis**

Prior antibiotic treatment

Fastidious organisms
    HACEK bacteria (*h*aemophilus, *a*ctinobacillus, *c*ardiobacterium, *e*ikenella, *k*ingella)
    Brucella species
    Legionella species
    Neisseria species
    Nocardia species

Intracellular bacteria
    Chlamydia
    Coxiella
    Bartonella
    Mycoplasma

Fungi
    Candida
    Aspergillus

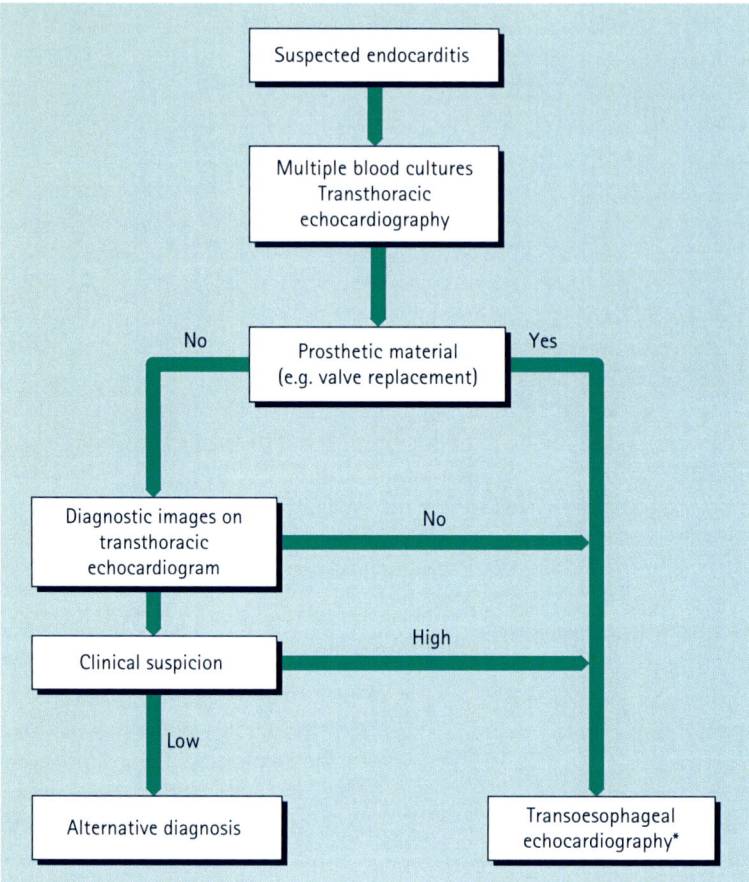

Figure 20.2 Diagnosis of infective endocarditis. *Repeat transoesophageal echocardiogram 48 hours if clinical suspicion is high (if the first transoesophageal echocardiogram is negative).

This showed significant deterioration in the aortic valve with severe aortic regurgitation. The patient subsequently underwent surgery to replace the aortic valve prosthesis. The indications for surgery in infective endocarditis are listed in Table 20.3.

Table 20.3 Indications for surgery

Native valve	Prosthetic valve
Stenosis or regurgitation resulting in heart failure	Stenosis or regurgitation resulting in heart failure
Infective endocarditis caused by fungal or highly resistant organisms	Endocarditis complicated by dehiscence of prosthetic valve
Endocarditis complicated by abscess formation, heart block, perforating or penetrating lesions (e.g. fistula)	Persistent or recurrent bacteraemia
Recurrent systemic emboli despite adequate medical therapy	Endocarditis complicated by abscess formation, heart block, perforating or penetrating lesions (e.g. fistula) Recurrent systemic emboli despite adequate medical therapy

Of note, despite the risk of embolic complications, anticoagulation is not routinely recommended in the treatment of endocarditis. However, patients with prosthetic valves are usually maintained on anticoagulation (warfarin may be replaced with intravenous heparin if surgical intervention is considered).

Recent Developments

The devastating complications of infective endocarditis, including significant risk of mortality (20% in some studies), have led to recommendations for antibiotic prophylaxis in patients perceived to be at risk of endocarditis (e.g. patients with prosthetic valves, some congenital heart disease and previous history of endocarditis). However, the subject of antibiotic prophylaxis is controversial with recent guidelines questioning the association between interventional procedure (dental and non-dental) and the development of infective endocarditis, the relative exposure to bacteraemia compared with regular toothbrushing, the effectiveness of antibiotic prophylaxis and the relative risk of anaphylaxis with antibiotic prophylaxis. The most recent guidelines issued by the National Institute of Clinical Excellence do *not* recommend routine antibiotic prophylaxis for preventing infective endocarditis.

Conclusion

Infective endocarditis is a potentially lethal condition. Definitive diagnosis requires microbiological evidence (multiple blood cultures) and evidence of endocardial involvement (transthoracic and/or transoesophageal echocardiography). Prolonged courses of bactericidal antibiotic treatment depending on the organism are usually required (particularly with prosthetic valve involvement) with surgical intervention in complicated cases.

Further Reading

Horstkotte D, Follath F, Gutschik E, *et al;* Task Force Members on Infective Endocarditis of the European Society of Cardiology; ESC Committee for Practice Guidelines (CPG); Document Reviewers. Guidelines on prevention, diagnosis and treatment of infective endocarditis executive summary; the task force on infective endocarditis of the European Society of Cardiology. *Eur Heart J* 2004; **25**: 267–76.

National Institute of Clinical Excellence. *Prophylaxis against Infective Endocarditis. Antimicrobial prophylaxis against infective endocarditis in adults and children undergoing interventional procedures.* March 2008.

Nishimura RA, Carabello BA, Faxon DP, *et al.* ACC/AHA 2008 guideline update on valvular heart disease: focused update on infective endocarditis: a report of the American College of Cardiology/American Heart Association Task Force on Practice Guidelines: endorsed by the Society of Cardiovascular Anesthesiologists, Society for Cardiovascular Angiography and Interventions, and Society of Thoracic Surgeons. *Circulation* 2008; **118**: 887–96.

Prendergast BD. Diagnostic criteria and problems in infective endocarditis. *Heart* 2004; **90**: 611–13.

SECTION FIVE

05

Cardiac Arrhythmias

21	Narrow complex tachycardia
22	Atrial fibrillation
23	Broad complex tachycardia
24	Bradyarrhythmia
25	Sudden cardiac death

PROBLEM

21 Narrow complex tachycardia

Case History

A 28-year-old man complained of intermittent palpitations about once a week. These palpitations were sometimes associated with breathlessness and did not appear to be related to physical activity. He has no past medical history. He is not on any regular medications and denies illicit drug use or excessive alcohol intake. There is no family history of sudden death. On examination, his regular resting heart rate was 60 beats/minute and blood pressure was 124/80 mmHg. Cardiovascular examination was unremarkable. His resting electrocardiogram (ECG) showed sinus rhythm with no evidence of pre-excitation and a normal QT interval.

How would you manage this man?

Background

Initial investigation should aim to identify the nature of the palpitations. Clinical history should distinguish whether the palpitations are regular or irregular, specific triggers, frequency, duration and the onset and termination (usually abrupt in arrhythmias). Supraventricular tachycardia often occurs in the absence of structural heart disease, but this should be carefully sought and excluded. An echocardiogram may be useful in this regard. Prognosis is generally more favourable in the absence of structural heart disease. The arrhythmia should be documented and this usually requires ambulatory monitoring. Twenty-four-hour holter monitoring may have only limited sensitivity if the palpitations occur only infrequently (on a weekly basis in this case). A loop recorder for 1 week may be appropriate. If a longer period of monitoring is required to document the arrhythmia, an implantable loop recorder (up to 3 years) may be considered. In this case, the patient-activated loop recorder documented a narrow complex tachycardia.

Subsequently, the patient presented to the emergency department with an episode of palpitations, and an ECG obtained at that time also documented a narrow complex tachycardia. The ECG (Figure 21.1) demonstrates a regular narrow complex tachycardia at a rate of 170 beats/minute. The P waves are not evident (probably buried within the QRS complexes). This is suggestive, although not diagnostic of atrioventricular nodal re-entry tachycardia (AVNRT). An AV re-entry tachycardia (AVRT) via a concealed accessory pathway is also a possibility and cannot always be differentiated from AVNRT based on surface ECG alone.

Almost all cases of narrow complex tachycardia represent supraventricular arrhythmia. The most common causes of supraventricular tachycardia are typical AVNRT and AVRT. Both AVNRT and AVRT, as the names suggest, involve a re-entry mechanism facilitated by two conduction pathways with different conduction properties. The AV node forms part of the re-entry circuit, while a second conduction pathway in the perinodal tissue or an accessory pathway form the other part of the circuit in AVNRT and AVRT respectively. The accessory pathway may or may not be concealed (based on evidence of pre-excitation on ECG during sinus rhythm). Pre-excitation on ECG reflects early ventricular activation by antegrade conduction via the accessory pathway, which bypasses the AV node, giving rise to the slurred upstroke (or downstroke) of the QRS complexes with a short PR interval (Figure 21.2). An example of pre-excitation is shown in Figure 21.2 with the typical short PR interval (due to rapid antegrade conduction via the accessory pathway bypassing the AV node) and slurring of the initial QRS (known as delta wave, which reflects early ventricular activation). The appearance of the delta wave

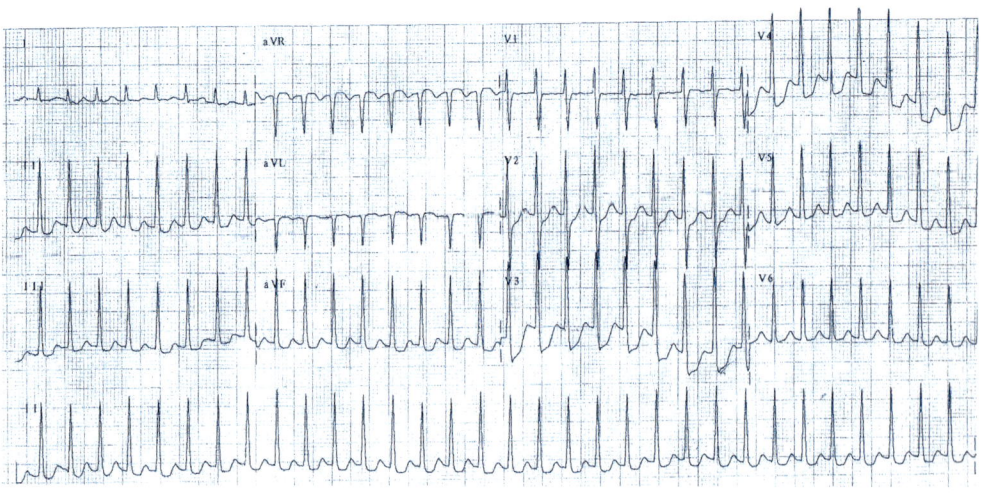

Figure 21.1 Narrow complex tachycardia.

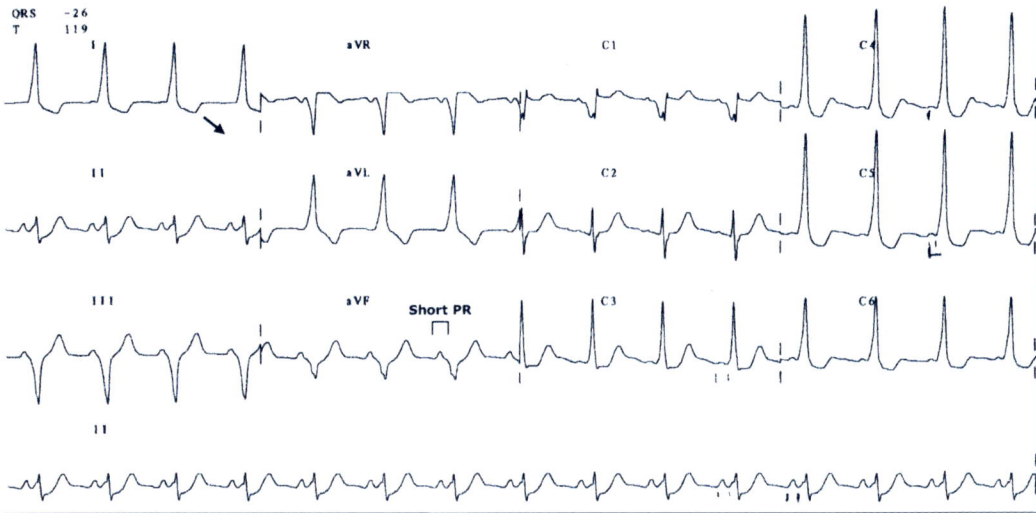

Figure 21.2 Ventricular pre-excitation on ECG.

will vary depending on the location of the accessory pathway. Wolff–Parkinson–White syndrome describes the association of clinical symptoms with supraventricular tachycardia and pre-excitation on the ECG. Figure 21.3 shows resolution of supraventricular tachycardia and reappearance of pre-excitation (delta wave) in sinus rhythm. Note, unlike the SVT in Figure 21.1 where there were no clear P waves, there are inverted retrograde P waves during tachycardia following the QRS complexes (arrows), which is more typical of AVRT than AVNRT.

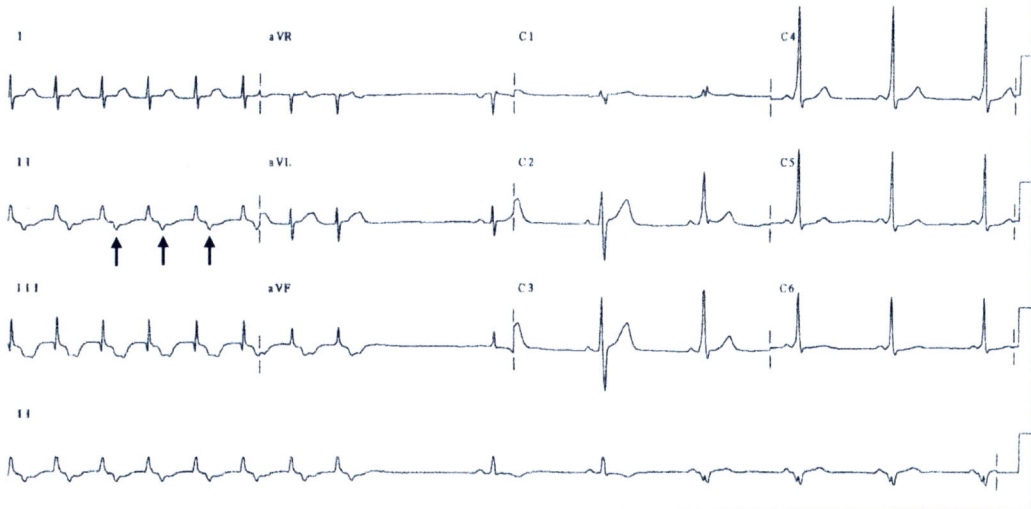

Figure 21.3 Termination of tachycardia and appearance of pre-excitation.

Other causes of supraventricular tachycardia include sinus node re-entry tachycardia, atrial tachycardia, paroxysmal junctional reciprocating tachycardia, atrial flutter and atrial fibrillation. In some cases, differentiating these different arrhythmias during tachycardia can be difficult as the changes may be subtle and may not be possible based on ECG alone. An example of typical atrial flutter with the 'saw-tooth' appearance is shown in Figure 21.4. Note, the flutter waves in typical atrial flutter are negative in the inferior leads and positive in lead V1.

At presentation, the patient's cardiorespiratory status should be assessed and, in the event of haemodynamic compromise, immediate electrical cardioversion is indicated. In the absence of haemodynamic compromise, vagal manoeuvres (e.g. carotid sinus massage) or intravenous adenosine may be used to terminate the arrhythmia. Both vagal manoeuvres and adenosine increase AV nodal conduction delay, thereby disrupting the re-entry circuit, which results in termination of the tachycardia. Other AV nodal-blocking agents such as β-blockers and non-dihydropyridine calcium channel blockers (verapamil and diltiazem) are also effective treatment for terminating supraventricular tachycardia, particularly AVNRT and AVRT (Figure 21.5). The heart rhythm should be recorded during administration of adenosine for the termination of the arrhythmia as useful diagnostic information may be obtained. In this case, the arrhythmia was terminated by intravenous adenosine.

Long-term treatment of recurrent supraventricular tachycardia depends on the arrhythmia itself. Radiofrequency ablation is a safe and effective treatment for AVNRT and AVRT with a success rate of over 90%. Successful ablation for AVNRT and AVRT is curative in most patients. Owing to the proximity to the AV node, radiofrequency ablation for AVNRT and AVRT (depending on the location of the accessory pathway) carries a small risk (generally <1%) of iatrogenic heart block, which may require a permanent pacemaker. Radiofrequency ablation is therefore recommended for patients with recurrent symptomatic AVNRT or AVRT, and particularly if the arrhythmia is poorly tolerated or there is associated pre-excitation of the ECG. This patient underwent a successful radiofrequency ablation procedure and remains free of palpitations.

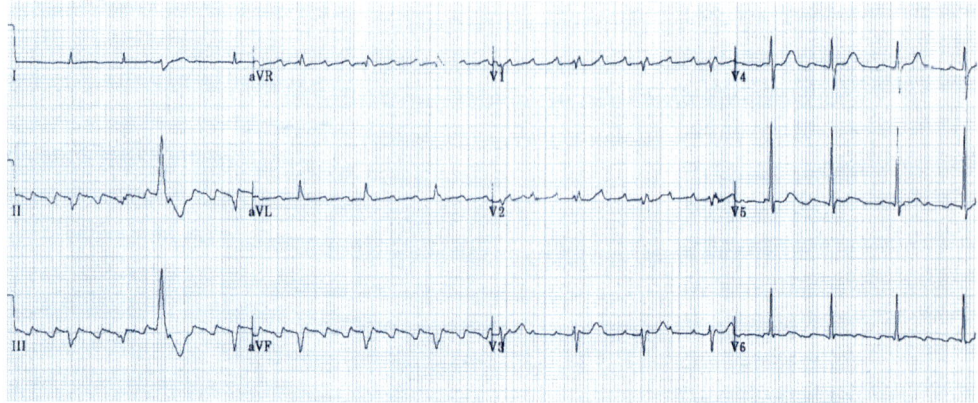

Figure 21.4 Atrial flutter.

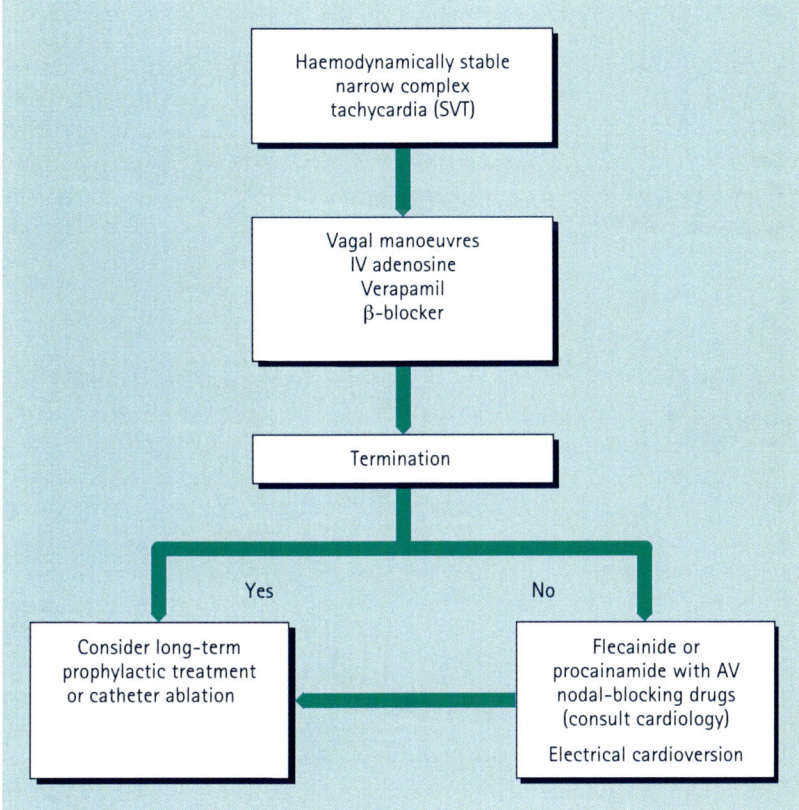

Figure 21.5 Management of narrow complex tachycardia. AV, atrioventricular; SVT, supraventricular tachycardia.

For patients with AVNRT who decline radiofrequency ablation, medical therapy with non-dihydropyridine calcium channel blockers or β-blockers may reduce the frequency of arrhythmia. Class I anti-arrhythmic agents such as flecainide and propafenone may be more effective and may be considered in patients with recurrent symptomatic episodes unresponsive to β-blockers and calcium channel blockers. Class III agents such as amiodarone and sotalol are rarely needed for the treatment of AVNRT, and in most cases may be inappropriate in view of the adverse effects and risk of pro-arrhythmia. In some cases, the conduction properties of the accessory pathway may deteriorate with age, which may lead to resolution of the re-entry pathway and arrhythmia.

Calcium channel blockers and digoxin may increase AV conduction delay and promote conduction via the accessory pathway. This may result in haemodynamic deterioration and should not be used as sole therapeutic agents in patients with AVRT and pre-excitation, particularly in the setting of atrial fibrillation with ventricular pre-excitation (i.e. atrial fibrillation with antegrade conduction via the accessory pathway). Flecainide and propafenone may be used in these cases and the addition of β-blockers may further reduce the frequency of symptomatic arrhythmia.

Recent Developments

In the LADIP (Loire-Ardèche-Drôme-Isère-Puy-de-Dôme) study, radiofrequency ablation was evaluated as first-line treatment following the first episode of symptomatic atrial flutter. This study included 102 patients and prospectively compared radiofrequency ablation against amiodarone therapy following first presentation of symptomatic atrial flutter. Radiofrequency ablation was associated with a significantly lower recurrence of atrial flutter compared with amiodarone (3.8% versus 29.5% over an average 13 months).

Conclusion

The most common causes of narrow complex tachycardia in younger patients are AVNRT and AVRT, the latter mediated by an accessory pathway. Differentiating the two conditions may not always be possible based on ECG alone. Structural heart disease is uncommon but should be excluded. The majority of these supraventricular tachycardias may be terminated by vagal manoeuvres, adenosine, β-blockers or verapamil. Radiofrequency ablation can achieve long-term cure in the majority of patients with AVNRT and AVRT with a small risk of iatrogenic heart block.

Further Reading

Blomström-Lunqvist C, Scheinman MM, Aliot EM, *et al.* ACC/AHA/ESC guidelines for the management of patients with supraventricular arrhythmias: a report of the American College of Cardiology/American Heart Association Task Force on Practice Guidelines and the European Society of Cardiology Committee for Practice Guidelines (Writing Committee to Develop Guidelines for the Management of Patients with Supraventricular Arrhythmias). *Circulation* 2003; **108**: 1871–909.

Da Costa A, Thévenin J, Roche F, *et al.*, for the Loire-Ardèche-Drôme-Isère-Puy-de-Dôme (LADIP) Trial of Atrial Flutter Investigators. Results from the Loire-Ardèche-Drôme-Isère-Puy-de-Dôme (LADIP) trial on atrial flutter, a multicentric prospective randomized trial comparing amiodarone and radiofrequency ablation after the first episode of symptomatic atrial flutter. *Circulation* 2006; **114**: 1676–81.

22 Atrial fibrillation

Case History

A 57-year-old man presented to the hospital following an episode of palpitations associated with breathlessness. On further inquiry, he gave a 6-month history of intermittent weekly palpitations, unrelated to exertion, lasting about 30 minutes each time. He has a long history of asthma but no known heart disease, hypertension or diabetes mellitus. On admission, his pulse was irregular with a heart rate ranging from 100 to 150 beats/minute with a blood pressure of 132/80 mmHg. Clinical examination was otherwise normal. His electrocardiogram (ECG) is shown in Figure 22.1.

What is the diagnosis?

How would you manage this patient?

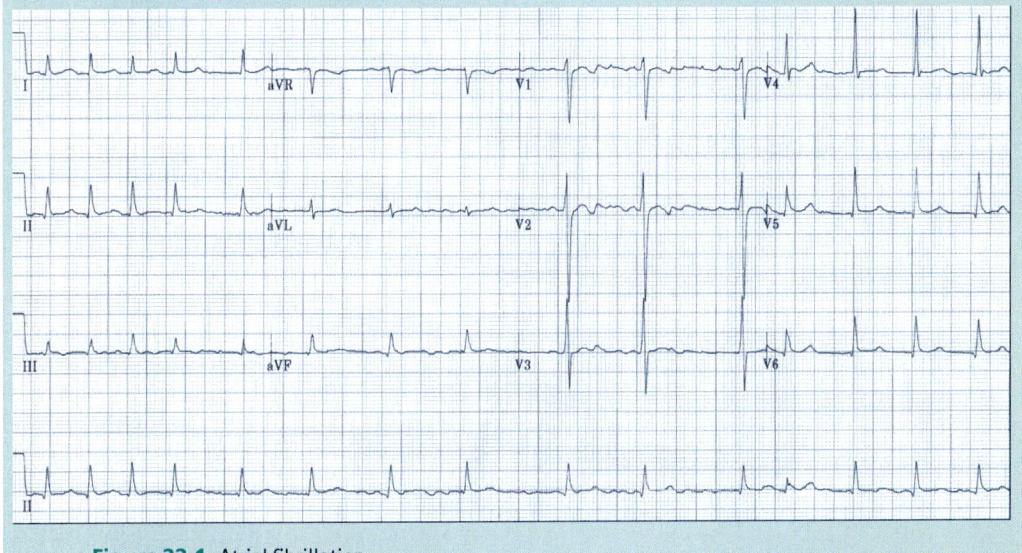

Figure 22.1 Atrial fibrillation.

Background

The electrocardiogram shows an irregular narrow complex tachycardia with no organ-ized P waves consistent with atrial fibrillation (AF). There is no electrocardiographic evidence of left ventricular hypertrophy or ischaemia. A clinical classification scheme based on consensus classifies AF on clinical presentation. New-onset AF may be classified as either paroxysmal (<7 days, usually <24 hours) or persistent (if sustained >7 days); and recurrent if more than two episodes. The classification of permanent AF is often arbitrary if cardioversion attempts are deemed unsuccessful or not pursued.

How would you manage this patient?

AF is frequently associated with underlying heart disease. For example, the prevalence of AF increases with the severity of heart failure. AF may also be precipitated by an acute illness (e.g. sepsis or surgery). Some causes and factors predisposing to AF are listed in Table 22.1. Clinical evaluation of a patient with new-onset AF should include thyroid function test, routine biochemistry and transthoracic echocardiogram (Figure 22.2) to exclude significant structural heart disease. Thyroid function test and ECG were both normal in this case.

In the absence of haemodynamic compromise when urgent cardioversion is indicated, the ventricular rate should be controlled as the initial treatment of this patient with

Table 22.1 Causes of atrial fibrillation

Myocardial disease
Valvular heart disease
Coronary artery disease
Congenital heart disease
Drugs and alcohol
Endocrine disorder (thyroid and phaeochromocytoma)
Postoperative and acute illness (e.g. sepsis)
Neurogenic (e.g. intracranial haemorrhage)
Idiopathic (lone)

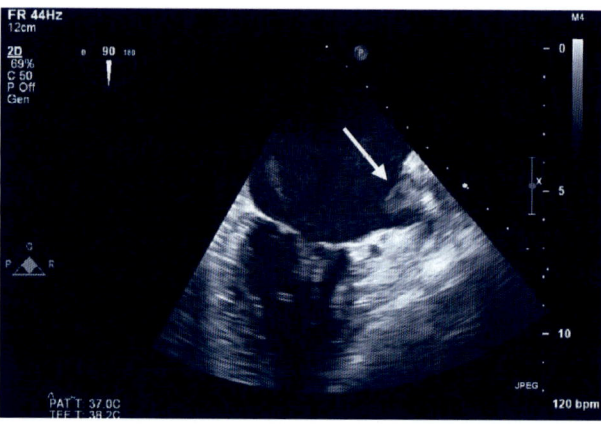

Figure 22.2 Thrombus in the left atrial appendage (arrow) on transoesophageal echocardiogram.

symptomatic AF. This is best achieved with atrioventricular (AV) nodal-blocking drugs such as β-blockers or non-dihydropyridine calcium channel antagonist (verapamil or diltiazem). Digoxin should not be considered the routine first-line rate-lowering drug, as the rate-lowering effects are inferior to β-blockers, diltiazem or verapamil. In particular, the sympathetic drive usually overwhelms the rate-lowering effect of digoxin, rendering it ineffective in patients during an acute illness. However, the addition of digoxin to β-blockers or calcium channel blockers may provide an additional rate-lowering effect, and may be considered if additional rate control is needed. Digoxin and amiodarone may also be appropriate in the setting of acute heart failure and hypotension when β-blockers and calcium channel antagonists may not be well tolerated. β-blockers are also contraindicated in the presence of asthma, as in this case. This patient was therefore commenced on verapamil.

Cardioversion may be performed to restore sinus rhythm in a patient with symptomatic AF (Figure 22.3). Direct current cardioversion (starting energy of 200 J, mono- or biphasic) under sedation or anaesthesia has a high success rate, although a significant

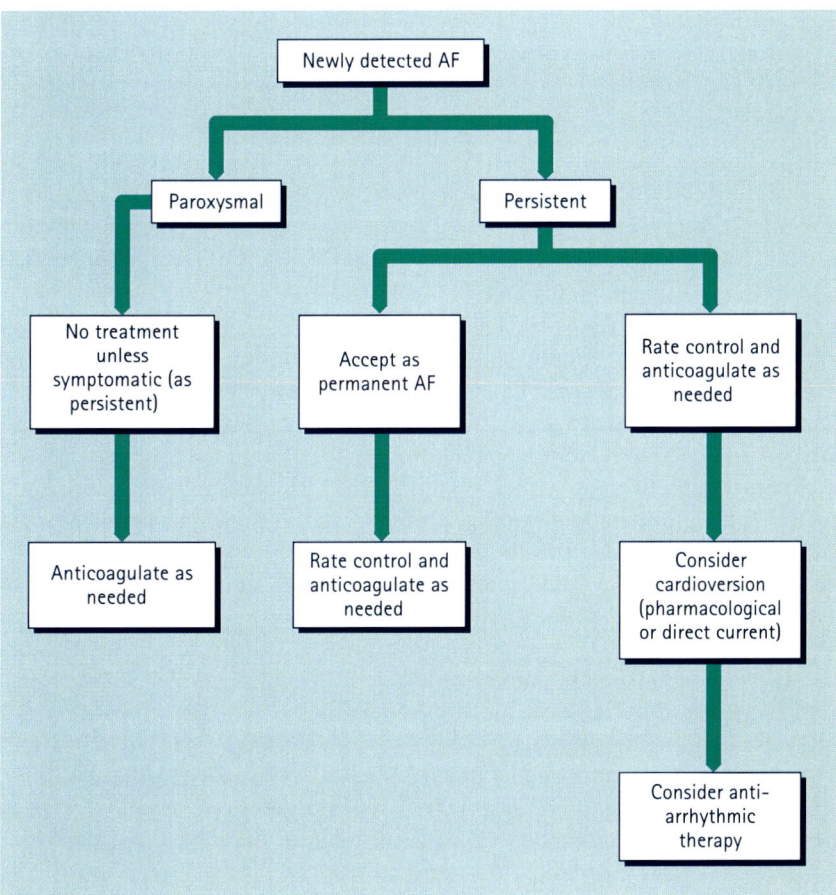

Figure 22.3 Management of newly detected atrial fibrillation (AF).

proportion of patients will experience early recurrence of the arrhythmia. Over 50% of patients will experience recurrence of AF in a year with the majority occurring in the first 2 weeks. Older patients with longer duration of AF and dilated left atrium or structural heart disease are more likely to have recurrence following cardioversion. The risks associated with direct current cardioversion are small and mainly related to thromboembolism and arrhythmia (e.g. sinus arrest and supraventricular tachycardia). The latter are usually transient.

Pharmacological cardioversion may be attempted as an alternative to direct current. While the risk of thromboembolism remains, irrespective of the cardioversion modality, pharmacological cardioversion obviates the need for sedation or anaesthesia. Pharmacological cardioversion, however, has a lower success rate compared with direct current cardioversion. Recommended agents for cardioversion are listed in Table 22.2. Pharmacological cardioversion with flecainide was considered in this patient but the patient reverted back into sinus rhythm spontaneously.

Table 22.2 Drugs for pharmacological cardioversion

Drug	Dose	Potential complications
Amiodarone	600–800 mg/day in divided doses until 10 g total, then 200–400 mg/day 300 mg then 1.2–1.8 g/day until 10 g (intravenous)	Bradycardia, QT prolongation, torsades de pointes (rare), phlebitis with intravenous use
Flecainide	200–300 mg/day 2 mg/kg up to 150 mg over 20 minutes (intravenous)	Hypotension, atrial flutter with rapid ventricular rate
Propafenone	600 mg 2 mg/kg over 20 minutes (intravenous)	Hypotension, atrial flutter with rapid ventricular rate

Cardioversion (whether by direct current or drugs) carries a risk of thromboembolism, particularly if the arrhythmia has been present for >48 hours. In a patient with AF for >48 hours, elective cardioversion should be deferred until 3 weeks of therapeutic anticoagulation has been instituted. Alternatively, a transoesophageal echocardiogram may be performed and cardioversion attempted in the absence of thrombus in the left atrial appendage. This transoesophageal echocardiogram-guided strategy has been shown to have comparable clinical outcomes compared with the conventional anticoagulation strategy. Anticoagulation should be continued for at least 4 weeks after cardioversion as recovery of atrial function may be delayed and can result in thromboembolism.

Long-term anticoagulation treatment should also be considered in patients with AF with the aim of preventing thromboembolic events. As the benefit of long-term anticoagulation is directly related to the absolute risk of thromboembolism, all patients with AF should be assessed for their risk of thromboembolism. One risk-stratification tool based on a number of clinical risk factors – congestive heart failure, hypertension, age >75 years, diabetes mellitus and a history of stroke or transient ischaemic attack – is the $CHADS_2$ score (Congestive heart failure, Hypertension, Age over 75, Diabetes, Stroke/TIA [2 points]) (Table 22.3). Anticoagulation should be considered in a patient with a score of 2 or more. Low-risk patients may be managed with aspirin. Hence, the patient in this case can be managed on aspirin. Of note, the decision for anticoagulation in paroxysmal AF should be considered in the same way as permanent AF.

Table 22.3 Risk stratification for thromboembolism

Congestive heart failure

Hypertension

Age >75 years

Diabetes mellitus

Stroke/transient ischaemic attack

1 point for each risk factor, except for stroke/TIA (2 points)
Anticoagulation recommended if score of 2 or more

The decision about long-term anti-arrhythmic treatment is dependent on the patient's symptoms. In patients with permanent AF who are asymptomatic, anti-arrhythmic drug treatment is not associated with improved outcomes compared with a rate control strategy with therapeutic anticoagulation. Indeed, even in patients with heart failure, in whom restoration of sinus rhythm may improve cardiac output, the use of amiodarone to maintain sinus rhythm has not been shown to improve clinical outcomes. Hence, long-term rate control with anticoagulation is a reasonable therapeutic strategy. Symptomatic patients may benefit (symptomatically) from anti-arrhythmic therapy, either taken regularly or in a 'pill in the pocket' (i.e. taken only when symptoms occur) approach in patients with infrequent attacks. Amiodarone has been shown to be more effective than sotalol in maintaining sinus rhythm, although long-term adverse effects are major concerns. Flecainide and propafenone have been used in a 'pill in the pocket' approach (concomitant use of AV nodal-blocking agents should be considered). Some anti-arrhythmic drugs for maintenance of sinus rhythm are listed in Table 22.4.

Table 22.4 Drugs for maintenance of sinus rhythm

Drug	Dose	Adverse effects
Amiodarone	100–400 mg/day	Photosensitivity, pulmonary and liver toxicity, thyroid dysfunction, neuropathy, eye complications, bradycardia
Disopyramide	400–750 mg/day	Torsades de pointes, dry eyes, dry mouth, urinary retention
Flecainide	200–300 mg/day	Ventricular arrhythmia, atrial flutter with rapid ventricular response, exacerbation of heart failure
Propafenone	450–900 mg/day	Ventricular arrhythmia, atrial flutter with rapid ventricular response, exacerbation of heart failure
Sotalol	160–320 mg/day	Torsade de pointes, bradycardia, bronchospasm

Radiofrequency ablation may be considered if anti-arrhythmic drugs fail to prevent or reduce the recurrence of symptomatic AF, but it is associated with peri-procedural risk of thromboembolism, cardiac tamponade and even mortality. Hence, radiofrequency ablation cannot yet be considered a first-line treatment option (Figure 22.4).

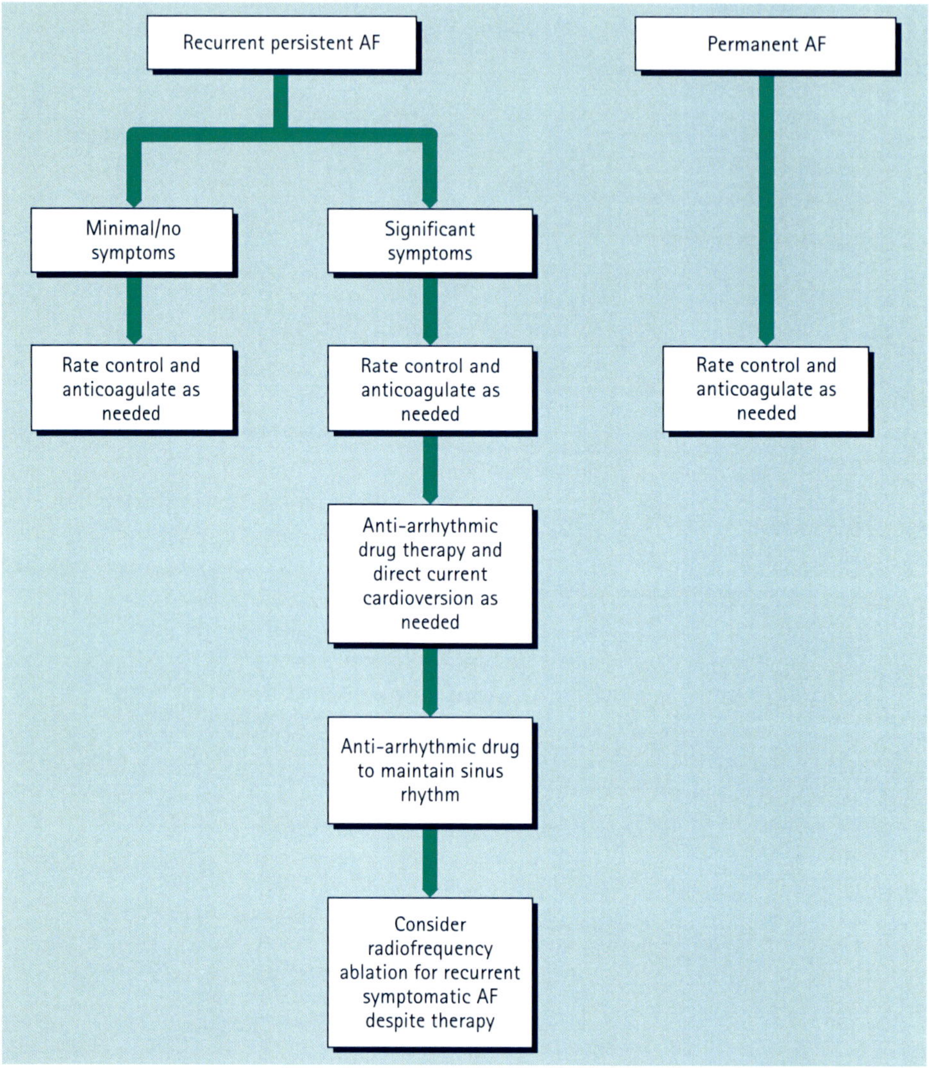

Figure 22.4 Management of recurrent atrial fibrillation (AF).

Recent Developments

Recent developments in the management of AF can be divided into new anti-arrhythmic drugs, non-pharmacological therapy and new anticoagulants. Dronedarone, a new non-iodinated amiodarone congener has Vaughan-Williams Class I-IV electrophysiological effects, but without significant thyroid or pulmonary toxicity. Dronedarone has been evaluated in a number of clinical trials. The ATHENA trial suggests that dronedarone may reduce the rates of hospitalisation in patients with AF. However, recent systematic analyses suggest that dronedarone may not be as effective as amiodarone in maintaining sinus rhythm in patients with AF. Other anti-arrhythmics with more specific activity in the atria (less risk of ventricular pro-arrhythmia) are currently being evaluated.

Radiofrequency ablation to electrically isolate the pulmonary veins is increasingly used for the treatment of AF (particularly paroxysmal AF) since the identification of 'triggers' originating from the pulmonary veins. The technique of AF ablation has evolved considerably over the last 10 years and continues to evolve rapidly with advances in electro-anatomical mapping, catheter design, ablation technology and greater understanding of the pathophysiological mechanisms in AF. Small, short-term randomised studies suggest that AF ablation may be superior to anti-arrhythmic drugs in the maintenance of sinus rhythm. Larger randomised trials are ongoing.

The recent Randomised evaluation of long-term anticoagulation therapy (RE-LY) study of over 18 000 patients with atrial fibrillation showed that dabigatran (a direct thrombin inhibitor) at a dose of 150 mg twice daily resulted in lower risk of stroke or systemic thromboembolism compared to warfarin with similar rates of major bleeding. Other novel anticoagulants such as rivaroxaban and apixaban (direct factor Xa inhibtor) are currently undergoing phase III clinical trials.

Conclusion

AF is the most common sustained arrhythmia. Newly detected AF should prompt a search for a potential cause, although this arrhythmia frequently occurs in the absence of significant structural heart disease, particularly in the younger population. In the absence of haemodynamic compromise, the ventricular rate may be controlled with AV nodal-blocking drugs and cardioversion (with anti-arrhythmic therapy to maintain sinus rhythm) may be considered for symptomatic patients. All patients should be considered for anticoagulation therapy based on the risk of thromboembolism.

Further Reading

Connolly SJ, Ezekowitz MD, Yusuf S, *et al*. Dabigatran versus warfarin in patients with atrial fibrillation. *N Engl J Med* 2009; **361**: 1139–51.

Fuster V, Rydén LE, Cannom DS, *et al.*; American College of Cardiology/American Heart Association Task Force on Practice Guidelines; European Society of Cardiology Committee for Practice Guidelines; European Heart Rhythm Association; Heart Rhythm Society. ACC/AHA/ESC 2006 Guidelines for the Management of Patients with Atrial Fibrillation: a report of the American College of Cardiology/American Heart Association Task Force on Practice Guidelines and the European Society of Cardiology Committee for Practice Guidelines (Writing Committee to Revise the 2001 Guidelines for the Management of Patients With Atrial Fibrillation): developed in collaboration with the European Heart Rhythm Association and the Heart Rhythm Society. *Circulation* 2006; **114**: e257–354.

Hohnloser SH, Crijns HJ, van Eickels M, *et al*. Effect of dronedarone on cardiovascular events in atrial fibrillation. *N Engl J Med* 2009; **360**: 668–78.

Lip GY and Tse HF. Management of atrial fibrillation. *Lancet* 2007; **370**: 604–18.

Noheria A, Kumar A, Wylie Jr JV, Josephson ME. Catheter ablation vs antiarrhythmic drug therapy for atrial fibrillation. A systematic review. *Arch Intern Med* 2008; **168**: 581–6.

Piccini JP, Hasselblad V, Peterson ED, *et al*. Comparative efficacy of dronedarone and amiodarone for the maintenance of sinus rhythm in patients with atrial fibrillation. *J Am Coll Cardiol* 2009; **54**: 1089–95.

PROBLEM

23 Broad complex tachycardia

Case History

A 68-year-old man presented to the emergency department feeling light-headed and 'slightly breathless', which started suddenly about 20 minutes ago. He denied any chest pain. He also gave a history of intermittent palpitations for the last month. These palpitations were sometimes associated with breathlessness but he had no significant breathlessness on exertion. He has a history of hypertension and an anterior myocardial infarction 5 years ago. The latter resulted in a reduced left ventricular ejection fraction of 35%. He takes ramipril, aspirin, simvastatin and bisoprolol. He denies illicit drug use or excessive alcohol intake. On examination, he had a regular resting heart rate of almost 200 beats/minute and blood pressure of 114/60 mmHg. His electrocardiogram (ECG) is shown in Figure 23.1. During examination, his systolic blood pressure dropped to 70 mmHg, necessitating emergency cardioversion.

What does the electrocardiogram show?

How would you manage this man?

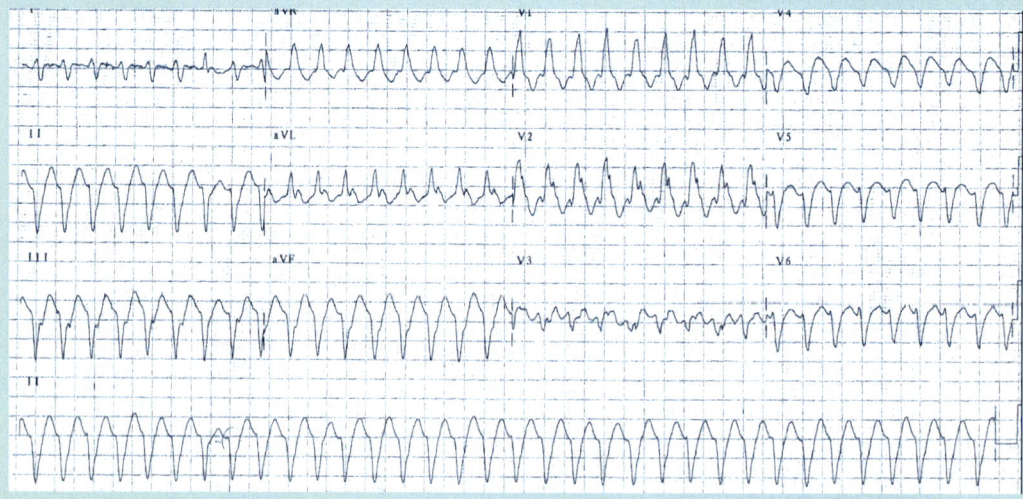

Figure 23.1 Broad complex tachycardia.

Background

 The ECG shows a regular broad complex tachycardia of almost 200 beats/minute. The frontal plane axis is superiorly directed with a right bundle branch block-type morphology. Broad complex tachycardia should be treated as ventricular tachycardia (VT) until proven otherwise. In this case, the electrocardiographic findings together with his background of myocardial infarction strongly suggest VT. The ECG following cardioversion shows evidence of previous anterior myocardial infarction.

How would you manage this man?

VTs can and often are life-threatening. The apparently 'normal' blood pressure should not trivialize this arrhythmia and haemodynamic deterioration can occur as in this case. Haemodynamic instability, generally defined as hypotension and evidence of impaired tissue perfusion should prompt immediate treatment to terminate the arrhythmia. This is best achieved by electrical cardioversion (synchronized to the R wave). The arrhythmia should not be interpreted as supraventricular in origin based on haemodynamic stability.

Termination of the arrhythmia should be followed by a search for potential substrates (e.g. scarring from previous myocardial infarction or cardiomyopathy) and triggers (e.g. electrolyte abnormalities or acute ischaemia) for ventricular arrhythmias. The ECG repeated after cardioversion may help identify these potential substrates (e.g. long QT interval) and triggers (e.g. ischaemia). Coronary angiography is also part of the routine assessment in many cases especially if there is evidence of myocardial ischaemia (e.g. ST elevation or significantly raised cardiac enzymes) or if coronary artery disease is probable, as coronary revascularization may reduce the risk of sudden death (Table 23.1). Of note, minor elevations in cardiac troponin may be evident in some cases, particularly if the episode of ventricular arrhythmia is prolonged in the presence of coronary artery

---

Table 23.1 ACC/AHA/ESC Class I recommendations

- Aggressive attempts should be made to treat heart failure that may be present in some patients with left ventricular dysfunction due to prior myocardial infarction and ventricular tachyarrhythmias.

- Aggressive attempts should be made to treat myocardial ischaemia that may be present in some patients with ventricular tachyarrhythmias.

- Coronary revascularization is indicated to reduce the risk of sudden cardiac death in patients with ventricular fibrillation when direct, clear evidence of acute myocardial ischaemia is documented to immediately precede the onset of ventricular fibrillation.

- If coronary revascularization cannot be carried out and there is evidence of prior myocardial infarction and significant left ventricular dysfunction, the primary therapy of patients resuscitated from ventricular fibrillation should be the implantable cardioverter defibrillator in patients who are receiving chronic optimal medical therapy and those who have reasonable expectation of survival with good functional status for more than 1 year.

- Implantable cardioverter defibrillator therapy is recommended for *primary* prevention to reduce total mortality by a reduction in sudden cardiac death in patients with left ventricular dysfunction due to prior myocardial infarction who are *at least 40 days post-myocardial infarction*, have a left ventricular ejection fraction less than or equal to 30–40%, are NYHA functional class II or III, are receiving chronic optimal medical therapy, and who have reasonable expectation of survival with a good functional status for more than 1 year.

- The implantable cardioverter defibrillator is effective therapy to reduce mortality by a reduction in sudden cardiac death in patients with left ventricular dysfunction due to prior myocardial infarction who present with haemodynamically unstable sustained ventricular tachycardia, are receiving chronic optimal medical therapy and who have reasonable expectation of survival with good functional status for more than 1 year.

disease and may not represent an ischaemic event precipitating ventricular arrhythmia. Therefore, interpretation of cardiac troponin should be individualized.

Cardiac imaging, generally with transthoracic echocardiography should form part of the routine assessment of a patient with ventricular arrhythmia. Cardiac magnetic resonance imaging, with greater image quality, is increasingly used, particularly in the assessment of cardiomyopathies. Ambulatory ECG recordings may be used when symptoms are sporadic and the diagnosis uncertain. Electrophysiological testing with intracardiac recordings and electrical stimulation is usually indicated only in a minority of patients when the diagnosis is uncertain and for the purpose of risk stratification.

In this case, the ECG following cardioversion showed evidence of anterior wall myocardial infarction. This patient underwent diagnostic coronary angiography, which confirmed a chronically occluded left anterior descending artery not amenable to revascularization. Left ventriculography confirmed significantly impaired left ventricular systolic function with akinesia of the anterior wall. A fixed defect was demonstrated on myocardial perfusion imaging consistent with his previous myocardial infarction. Serum electrolytes and subsequent cardiac enzymes, including troponin, were all within normal limits, providing further evidence that this event was not a result of an acute myocardial infarction.

β-blockers are indicated in patients with impaired left ventricular systolic function and heart failure, even in the absence of ventricular arrhythmias. These drugs are safe and effective anti-arrhythmic agents and have been shown to reduce the risk of sudden cardiac deaths in patients with heart failure. Therefore, β-blockers should be considered the mainstay of anti-arrhythmic therapy. However, the use of other anti-arrhythmic agents in patients with heart failure may be complicated by pro-arrhythmia, negative inotropic effects and adverse (non-cardiac) effects, which may be associated with adverse clinical outcomes. For these reasons, sodium channel blockers (class I anti-arrhythmic agents) and sotalol (class III agent) are generally contraindicated in patients with heart failure.

Amiodarone has been shown to have a neutral effect on survival in patients with heart failure although an analysis of the SCD-HeFT study (Sudden Cardiac Death in Heart Failure Trial) suggested potential harm in patients with New York Heart Association III heart failure and ejection fraction of <35%. As the adverse effects of amiodarone accumulate with increasing duration of therapy, it should be avoided if possible in younger patients. Hence, routine use of amiodarone in patients with heart failure is not recommended. Amiodarone may be considered in specific cases (see below) particularly in conjunction with an implantable cardioverter defibrillator (ICD).

The use of ICDs has been shown in a number of clinical trials to have improved survival in patients with haemodynamically significant ventricular arrhythmias (i.e. secondary prevention against sudden death) and patients with significantly impaired left ventricular systolic function due to ischaemic heart disease (and non-ischaemic cardiomyopathy to a lesser extent) even in the absence of sustained ventricular arrhythmia (i.e. primary prevention) (Table 23.2). Hence, ICDs are indicated in patients with sustained symptomatic or haemodynamically significant ventricular arrhythmias in the absence of reversible causes (Figure 23.2).

Current ICDs are capable of pacing for bradycardia (as in conventional pacemakers), pacing for VT (anti-tachycardia pacing), synchronized shock (cardioversion) or defibrillation. Inappropriate arrhythmia detection (e.g. detection of atrial tachycardia as ventricular arrhythmia), which can lead to inappropriate therapy, including shocks, remains the major limitation of implantable defibrillators and is clearly undesirable.

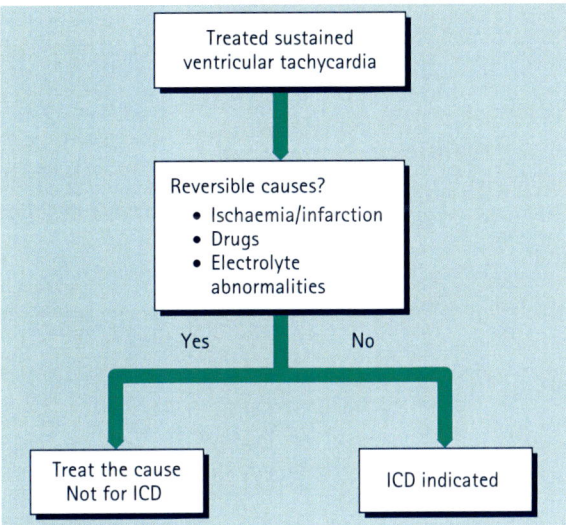

Figure 23.2 ICD in patients with sustained ventricular tachycardia. ICD, implantable cardioverter defibrillator.

Table 23.2 ICD in primary prevention

Study	n	Study criteria	Results
MADIT	196	EF≤35% (ischaemic) MI>3 weeks before study Inducible VT on EPS Asymptomatic NSVT NYHA I-III	Relative risk 0.25 (0.07–0.83)
MADIT II	1232	MI>1 month before study EF≤30% (ischaemic) NYHA I-III	Relative risk 0.39 (0.24–0.61)
SCD-HEFT	2521	EF≤35% NYHA II-III (versus amiodarone or placebo)	52% ischaemic cardiomyopathy Relative risk 0.77 (0.62–0.96)

MADIT, Multicenter Automatic Defibrillator Implantation Trial; SCD-HEFT, Sudden Cardiac Death in Heart Failure Trial; EPS, electrophysiological study; NSVT, non-sustained ventricular tachycardia; EF, ejection fraction; NYHA, New York Heart Association.

Programming of discrimination algorithms in the ICD should reduce the incidence of inappropriate therapy but in some cases concomitant anti-arrhythmic therapy (including amiodarone) may be required to control atrial arrhythmias. The combination of β-blocker and amiodarone may also be indicated in patients with recurrent sustained ventricular arrhythmias associated with frequent shocks from ICDs. Chest radiographs of an ICD and pacemaker are shown in Figure 23.3 for comparison.

The man in this case has significant left ventricular impairment secondary to ischaemic heart disease and haemodynamically significant ventricular arrhythmia, not caused by acute myocardial infarction. Hence, an ICD is indicated for secondary prevention, and a dual chamber ICD was implanted without complications. He was eventually discharged on a full dose of bisoprolol (without amiodarone).

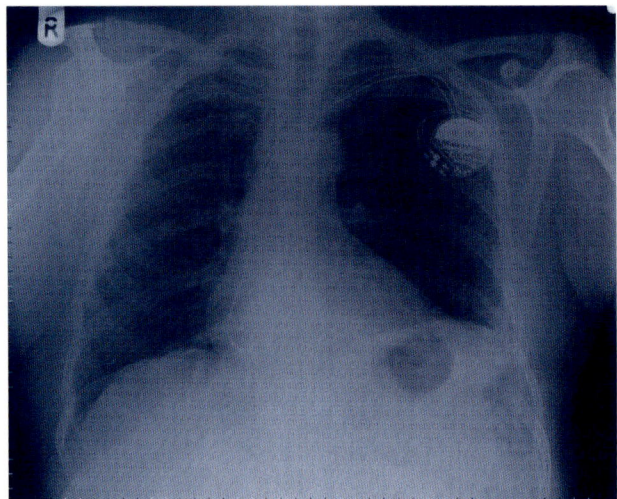

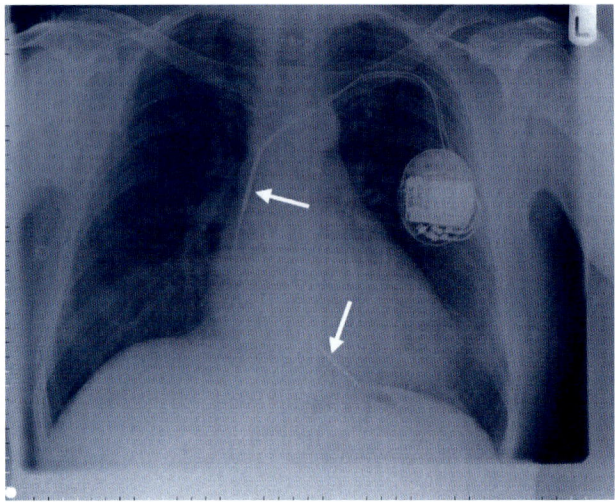

Figure 23.3 Pacemaker (A) compared with an implantable cardioverter defibrillator (ICD) (B). Note the larger device and thicker leads with the ICD due to the need for high-voltage shock coils (arrows).

In some cases, VT may be associated with a structurally normal heart. One example is the VT originating from the right ventricular outflow tract. These VTs typically have a left bundle branch block morphology with an inferiorly directed frontal plane axis (Figure 23.4). Radiofrequency ablation can cure patients with right ventricular outflow tract VT and it should be considered the treatment of choice.

Recent Developments

 ICDs are currently the treatment of choice in patients with life-threatening ventricular arrhythmia, particularly in the setting of left ventricular dysfunction associated with

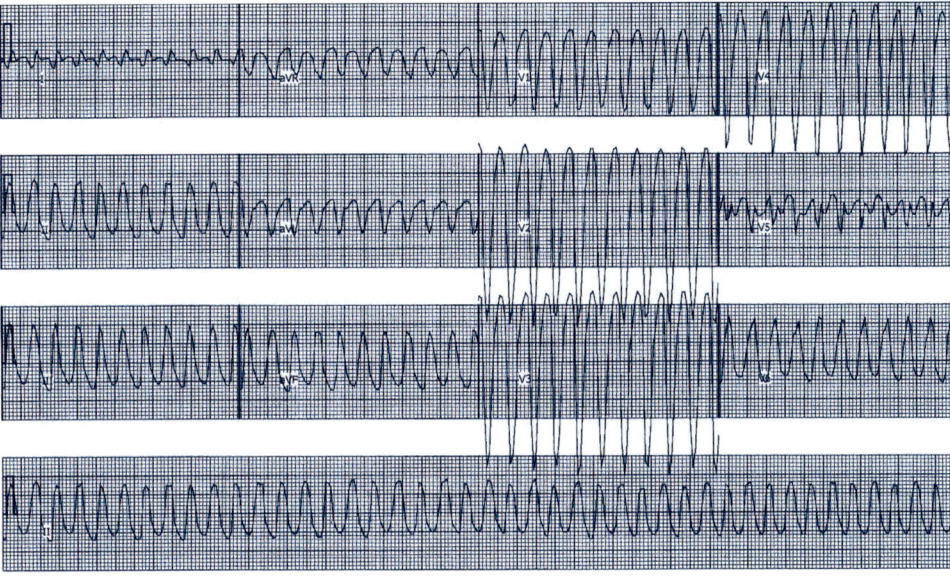

Figure 23.4 Right ventricular outflow tract VT with left bundle branch morphology and inferiorly directed axis.

coronary artery disease. Radiofrequency ablation of VT has recently been shown to reduce the need for ICD shocks or therapies. Ablation of VT may be considered in patients complicated by frequent recurrent VT.

Conclusion

Broad complex tachycardia should be treated as ventricular in origin until proven otherwise. Haemodynamic deterioration may occur, sometimes precipitously, and it should be treated with immediate electrical cardioversion. Potential substrates (e.g. ischaemic heart disease and cardiomyopathy) and triggers (e.g. acute myocardial infarction) should be identified and treated. ICDs are indicated for secondary prevention in patients with haemodynamically significant ventricular arrhythmia without reversible causes (e.g. electrolyte abnormalities or acute myocardial infarction) or primary prevention in patients without previous sustained ventricular arrhythmias but at risk of life-threatening ventricular arrhythmias because of significant structural heart disease.

Further Reading

Epstein AE, DiMarco JP, Ellenbogen KA, Estes, *et al*. ACC/AHA/HRS2008 guidelines for device-based therapy of cardiac rhythm abnormalities: executive summary: a report of the American College of Cardiology/American Heart Association Task Force on Practice Guidelines (Writing Committee to Revise the ACC/AHA/NASPE 2002 Guideline Update for Implantation of Cardiac Pacemakers and Antiarrhythmia Devices). *Circulation* 2008; **117**: 2820–40.

European Heart Rhythm Association; Heart Rhythm Society, Zipes DP, Camm AJ, Borggrefe M, et al; American College of Cardiology; American Heart Association Task Force; European Society of Cardiology Committee for Practice Guidelines. ACC/AHA/ESC 2006 guidelines for management of patients with ventricular arrhythmias and the prevention of sudden cardiac death: a report of the American College of Cardiology/American Heart Association Task Force and the European Society of Cardiology Committee for Practice Guidelines (Writing Committee to Develop Guidelines for Management of Patients With Ventricular Arrhythmias and the Prevention of Sudden Cardiac Death). *J Am Coll Cardiol* 2006; **48**: e247–346.

PROBLEM

24 Bradyarrhythmia

Case History

 An 81-year-old woman presented with 2 weeks of worsening shortness of breath and dizziness on exertion. She has a history of hypertension and bioprosthetic aortic valve replacement surgery the year before for degenerative calcific aortic stenosis. She is on ramipril, aspirin and simvastatin. On examination, her pulse was irregular at 40 beats/minute, with a blood pressure of 110/62 mmHg. Careful observation of her jugular vein indicated intermittent prominent 'pulsations'. She had mild peripheral oedema but clinical examination was otherwise normal. Her electrocardiogram (ECG) is shown in Figure 24.1.

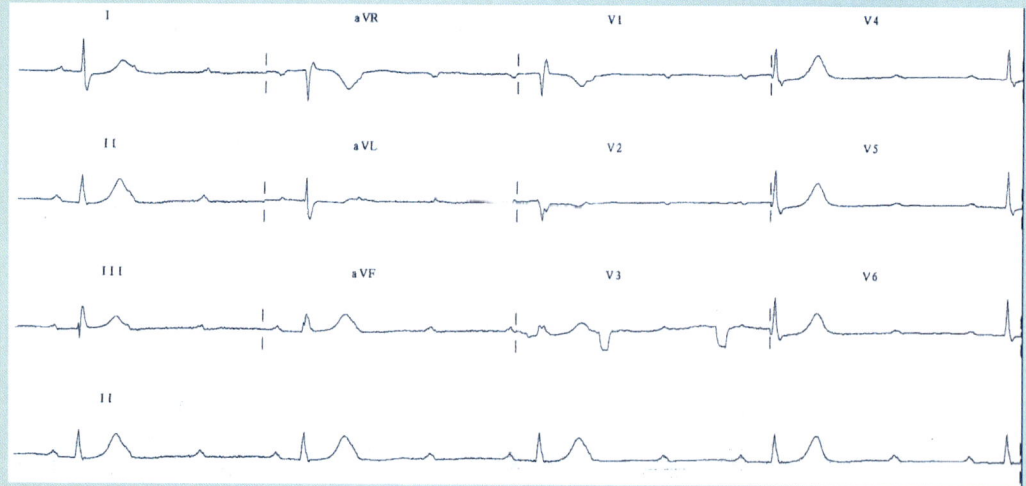

Figure 24.1 Complete heart block.

24 Bradyarrhythmia

What does the electrocardiogram show?

What is the likely cause of the slow heart rhythm?

How would you manage this patient?

Background

The ECG shows regular P waves with no consistent relationship with the QRS complexes (i.e. atrioventricular [AV] dissociation). The underlying ventricular rate is about 40 beats/minute with narrow QRS complexes suggestive of incomplete right bundle branch block. The level of conduction block cannot always be determined from surface ECGs although escape rhythms with broad QRS complexes are suggestive of conduction block below the AV node.

What is the likely cause of the slow heart rhythm?

Her background history of calcific aortic valve disease and valve replacement surgery is likely to be relevant. The association between aortic valve surgery and conduction tissue abnormality is well documented. The close proximity to the aortic valve exposes the AV node and conduction tissue to the risk of damage either from the valve disease (calcification) itself or at the time of aortic valve surgery. Degenerative changes in the conduction tissue may also contribute to her rhythm abnormality. Thyroid dysfunction, drug toxicity (e.g. β-blockers and verapamil) and electrolyte abnormalities (e.g. hyperkalaemia) should be excluded in all cases and should be part of the routine assessment of a patient with bradyarrhythmia. The clinical history and ECG should also be scrutinized for evidence of myocardial infarction. This patient did not give any history suggestive of ischaemia and was not on any rate-lowering medications.

How would you manage this patient?

The patient's cardiorespiratory stability should form the initial assessment of a patient with bradyarrhythmia. Intravenous atropine and temporary pacing may be instituted in a patient with significant haemodynamic compromise, recurrent syncope at rest and patients with tachyarrhythmias secondary to bradyarrhythmia. The anticholinergic effect of atropine antagonizes the vagal inhibitory effects on AV nodal conduction and is effective particularly if the conduction block is located at the level of the AV node. Atropine may not, however, reverse bradyarrhythmia due to distal (in the His–Purkinje system) conduction tissue disease and may even exacerbate conduction block. Aminophylline has also been used in the past for its antagonistic effects on adenosine, but was found not to be effective in bradyarrhythmic cardiac arrests. Aminophylline may even be pro-arrhythmic.

Temporary cardiac pacing is conventionally achieved by an external pacing system using external pacing pads or insertion of a transvenous (endocardial) temporary pacing wire, although epicardial and gastro-oesophageal approaches are well described. The indications for temporary cardiac pacing are listed in Table 24.1. External or transcutaneous pacing can be achieved rapidly and it requires only minimal training. External pacing, however, may be distressing for the patient as it induces muscular contractions and

Table 24.1 Indications for temporary pacing
Bradycardia associated with acute myocardial infarction 　Asystole 　Symptomatic (hypotension) bradycardia unresponsive to atropine 　Bilateral bundle branch block 　New or indeterminate age bifascicular block with first-degree heart block 　Mobitz type II second-degree atrioventricular block or complete heart block*
Bradycardia not associated with acute myocardial infarction 　Asystole 　Second- or third-degree AV block with haemodynamic compromise 　Ventricular tachyarrhythmia secondary to bradycardia
*Atrioventricular block may be transient in patients with inferior myocardial infarction and temporary pacing may be withheld if haemodynamically stable.

in most cases requires sedation if the patient is conscious. Hence, external pacing should be considered as a 'bridge' to transvenous temporary pacing. Epicardial and oesophageal approaches are not generally used in emergency settings in the emergency department.

The choice of vascular access site for temporary transvenous pacing may be largely dictated by the experience of the operator, but the right internal jugular vein offers the most direct route and has the highest success rate and lowest complication rates. A temporary pacing wire in the femoral vein limits patient mobility and predisposes to infection and venous thromboembolism, and should be avoided if possible. The subclavian veins should be avoided if there is concomitant anticoagulation therapy and the left subclavian vein in particular should be avoided, as this is often the site for the permanent pacemaker system. Complications may occur particularly in inexperienced hands and may be related to vascular access (e.g. haematoma, infection and pneumothorax) or the pacing lead (e.g. arrhythmias, lead displacement with loss of capture and ventricular perforation). In this case, temporary pacing was not indicated and she was monitored before receiving a permanent pacemaker the next day.

The nomenclature for permanent pacemakers is listed in Table 24.2. Dual chamber pacing refers to a pacing lead in the right atrium and the right ventricle, while single chamber pacemakers may have the pacing lead either in the right atrium or the right ventricle. Clinical trials comparing single chamber ventricular and dual chamber pacemakers in AV conduction disease have not shown significant survival benefit with dual chamber pacemaker systems. However, there appears to be a lower risk of atrial fibrillation and stroke with dual chamber pacemakers, particularly if the pacemaker is implanted for sinus node disease. Single chamber ventricular pacing results in the loss of

Table 24.2 Pacemaker nomenclature			
1st letter: Chamber paced	2nd letter: Chamber sensed	3rd letter: Mode of response to sensed beat	4th letter: Programmable rate response
A: atrium	A: atrium	I: inhibits pacing output	R if rate response available
V: ventricle	V: ventricle	T: triggers pacing output	
D: dual chamber	D: dual chamber	D: dual	

atrioventricular synchrony (dissociation of atrial and ventricular beats), which may result in the pacemaker syndrome. Symptoms of the pacemaker syndrome may consist of dizzy spells, syncope, chest discomfort, shortness of breath and palpitations and may be resolved by upgrading from a single to dual chamber pacemaker. The incidence of pacemaker syndrome ranges from about 5% to almost 30% depending on the study.

The choice of permanent pacemaker is dependent on a number of factors, but particularly the indication for permanent pacing itself (Figure 24.2). Single chamber ventricular pacemakers are indicated in patients with permanent atrial fibrillation and conduction block, as atrial fibrillation precludes any effective atrial pacing. Single chamber atrial pacemakers may be indicated in patients with sinus node disease without conduction disease at the AV node or more distally. However, patients with AV nodal conduction disease in addition to the sinus node disease will require a dual chamber pacemaker. Dual chamber pacemakers are generally indicated in AV conduction block, as in this case. Commonly used pacing modes are DDD(R), which maintains atrial and ventricular synchrony, VVI(R) and AAI(R) in single chamber atrial and ventricular pacemakers respectively. The letter 'R' refers to rate response, which may be useful in patients with chronotropic incompetence (inability to increase heart rate in response to exertion).

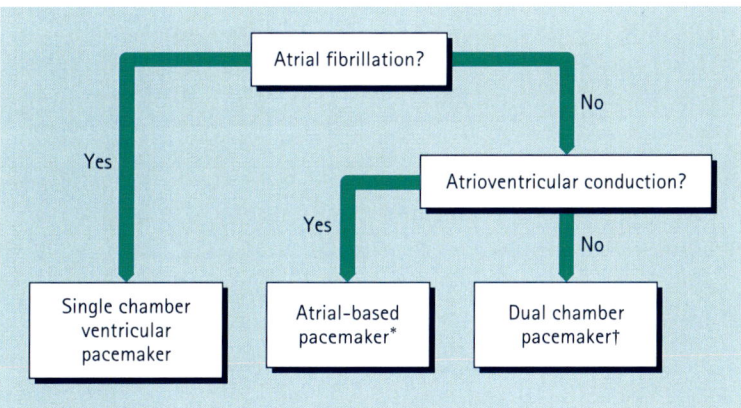

Figure 24.2 Factors affecting the choice of permanent pacemaker. *Single chamber atrial pacemaker if intact atrioventricular conduction, absence of ventricular conduction delay (narrow QRS) and Wenckebach point over 100 beats/minute. Alternatively, dual chamber pacemaker with algorithms to minimize ventricular pacing. †Note, no mortality benefit over single chamber ventricular pacemaker in elderly patients with atrioventricular conduction disease.

Recent Development

Pacemaker treatment has been evaluated in a number of studies over the last few years. The UK PACE study (Promoting Healthy Ageing with Cognitive Exercise) of elderly patients with AV heart block compared dual chamber versus single chamber ventricular pacemakers and reported no significant difference in overall survival. However, single chamber ventricular pacemakers in the setting of sinus node disease are associated with a higher risk of atrial fibrillation and stroke compared with dual chamber pacemakers. Furthermore, based on post-hoc analyses of clinical trials, high frequency of right ventricular pacing in patients with dual chamber pacemakers is related to a higher risk of atrial fibrillation and heart failure. This has led to the development of new pacemaker algorithms to minimize right ventricular pacing (in patients with sinus node disease). Indeed, the SAVE PACE (Search AV Extension and Managed Ventricular Pacing for Promoting Atrioventricular Conduction) study demonstrated a lower incidence of atrial fibrillation with the reduction in frequency of right ventricular pacing.

Conclusion

Patients presenting with bradyarrhythmia should be carefully assessed for haemodynamic compromise. Atropine may be effective in some cases but temporary cardiac pacing may be required in the majority of patients with significant haemodynamic compromise. Insertion of a permanent pacemaker is indicated in the absence of reversible causes (e.g. electrolyte abnormalities or drug toxicity) and dual chamber pacemakers are generally recommended in patients with AV conduction disease.

Further Reading

Fitzpatrick A, Sutton R. A guide to temporary pacing. *BMJ* 1992; **304**: 365–9.

Trohman RG, Kim MH, Pinski SL. Cardiac pacing: state-of-the-art. *Lancet* 2004; **364**: 1701–19.

PROBLEM

25 Sudden cardiac death

Case History

A 56-year-old man with a history of chronic obstructive pulmonary disease presented with worsening of breathlessness associated with a cough producing yellow–green sputum. He has a history of hypertension treated with bendroflumethiazide but no known heart disease. On admission, he was treated with nebulized bronchodilators (β-agonists) and a combination of amoxicillin and erythromycin. He complained of some palpitations the next day and the admitting physician noted a brief run of ventricular tachycardia on the monitor. An electrocardiogram (ECG) was performed, which is shown in Figure 25.1. He was transferred to the cardiac care unit where the ventricular arrhythmia (Figure 25.1) was documented before he suffered a cardiac arrest.

What is the diagnosis?

What is the cause of his arrhythmia?

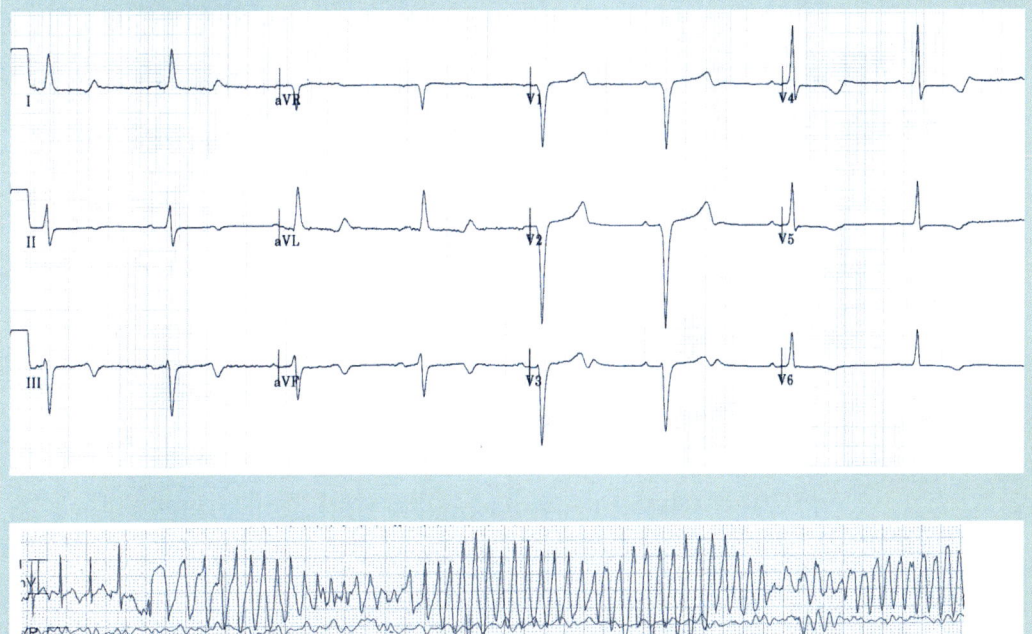

Figure 25.1 QT prolongation (top) and Torsades de Pointes (bottom).

Background

The ECG showed a sinus rhythm with a prolonged QT interval when corrected for heart rate. The ventricular arrhythmia is a polymorphic ventricular tachycardia. Hence, this man suffered torsades de pointes related to prolongation of his QT interval.

QT interval represents ventricular depolarization and repolarization. This interval should be measured from the beginning of the QRS to the end of the T wave. The 12-lead ECG should be carefully examined to identify the lead that clearly shows the end of the T wave (usually leads II and V5). QT intervals measured by computerized algorithms may provide rapid assessment but may also be prone to measurement error/variability and may not be reliable. As QT interval varies with heart rate (longer during bradycardia and shorter with increase in heart rate), the QT interval should be corrected for heart rate. There are a number of formulas for heart rate correction and all have limitations, but the Bazett formula is generally used. The Bazett formula ($QTc = QT/\sqrt{RR}$) uses 'seconds' instead of 'milliseconds' as the unit of measurement. A corrected QT interval of 450 ms in men and 460 ms in women is conventionally regarded as the upper limit of normal as these cut-offs represent the top 1% of the population.

What is the cause of his arrhythmia?

This man was successfully resuscitated. On reviewing his biochemistry, he was noted to have significant hypokalaemia (2.4 mmol/l) and hypomagnesaemia, probably due to the thiazide diuretic and nebulized β-agonists. These electrolyte abnormalities contribute to prolongation of the QT interval. However, a large number of medications also have well documented effects on the QT interval, including macrolide antibiotics (erythromycin). Medications with documented QT prolongation effects are listed in Table 25.1. The use of multiple drugs with QT prolonging effects increases the risk of arrhythmia further. Hence, QT interval should be carefully assessed (at peak plasma concentration) when the use of a drug with QT prolonging effects is considered.

Table 25.1 Drugs associated with prolongation of QT interval

Antiarrhythmics
   Sotalol
   Quinidine
   Procainamide
   Disopyramide

Antipsychotics
   Thioridazine
   Olanzapine
   Risperidone

Antidepressants
   Amitriptyline
   Imipramine
   Sertraline
   Venlafaxine

Antibiotics/anti-infectives
   Erythromycin
   Gatifloxacin
   Ketoconazole

Following successful resuscitation, the electrolyte abnormalities were corrected and erythromycin was discontinued. A subsequent ECG confirmed normalization of the corrected QT interval with no further ventricular arrhythmias. An implantable cardioverter defibrillator is not indicated in this case, as there was a clear reversible cause for the ventricular arrhythmia.

Prolongation of the QT interval may also be a result of inherited ion (particularly potassium and sodium) channel abnormalities. Unlike the man in this case, those individuals with congenital long QT syndromes may present dramatically with syncope and sudden death as the initial presentation. Indeed, congenital long QT syndromes are characterized by prolongation of the QT interval, syncope, 'seizures' and sudden death due to ventricular arrhythmias (torsade de pointes) in apparently healthy children and young adults. Some cases of sudden infant deaths have been attributed to congenital long QT syndrome. The prognosis and triggers of sudden cardiac death in patients with congenital long QT syndrome are related to the QT interval and the genotype. Hence, knowledge of the genotype may improve the management of these patients. These patients should be managed in specialist clinics by a multidisciplinary team, including a cardiologist with specialist experience and individuals with expertise in clinical genetics.

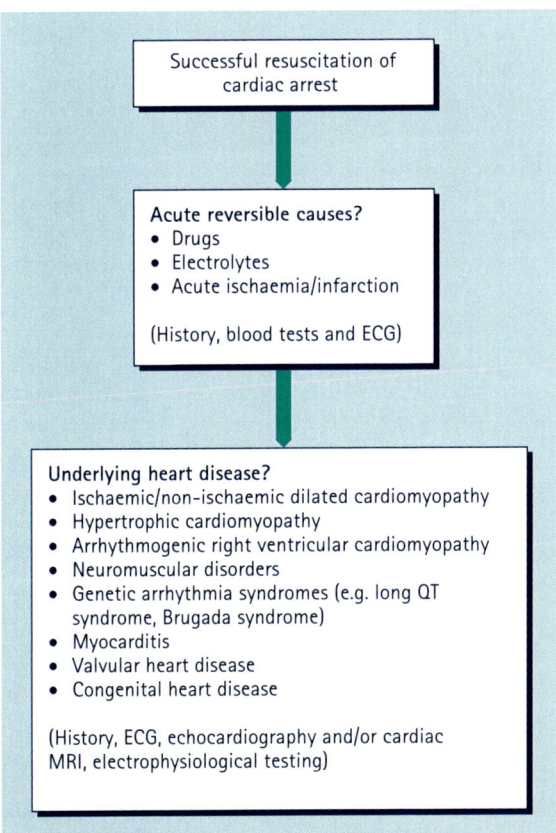

Figure 25.2 Investigation of sudden cardiac death. ECG, electrocardiogram; MRI, magnetic resonance imaging.

Other sudden death syndromes include catecholaminergic polymorphic ventricular tachycardia, hypertrophic cardiomyopathy, familial dilated cardiomyopathy with atrioventricular block, Brugada syndrome and arrhythmogenic right ventricular dysplasia. Catecholaminergic polymorphic ventricular tachycardia is a malignant condition characterized by ventricular tachycardia induced by exertion or emotion (Figure 25.2). β-blockers are ineffective in a significant proportion of cases and an implantable cardioverter defibrillator may be indicated. Familial dilated cardiomyopathy and atrioventricular block is characterized by cardiomyocyte death and atrioventricular nodal/bundle branch conduction abnormality. These patients are at increased risk of sudden death even with cardiac pacing and an implantable cardioverter defibrillator may be indicated.

Brugada syndrome is characterized by ST elevation in the precordial leads and risk of sudden cardiac death. Arrhythmogenic right ventricular dysplasia is characterized by fibrofatty replacement predominantly of the right ventricle and ventricular arrhythmias. Clinical diagnosis is difficult and genetic testing is only recommended for cascade screening of relatives. These sudden death syndromes should be managed in specialist multidisciplinary clinics due to the complexity in terms of diagnosis and treatment for the individual and the family.

Recent Developments

The sudden death of high profile athletes has generated much debate and controversy about screening for occult cardiomyopathy or sudden death syndromes. Some countries require electrocardiograms in addition to clinical history and examination for their athletes prior to training and competition (a position endorsed by the Lausanne recommendations for the International Olympic Committee) but routine 12-lead ECG is not recommended by the American Heart Association as part of the pre-competition screening (only if the athletes fail the initial clinical assessment).

A large series reported by Pelliccia *et al.* found electrocardiographic abnormalities (mainly T-wave changes) in 123 of 12 550 athletes screened (about 1%). Of these 123 athletes, 39 were found to have cardiac abnormalities (most commonly hypertrophic cardiomyopathy) on further investigation. Of the remaining 84 athletes, three did not undergo repeat assessment. Among the 81 athletes with follow-up assessment (average follow-up of 9 years), 11 developed cardiomyopathy or other cardiovascular abnormalities (including hypertension and coronary artery disease) but the remaining 70 did not develop a cardiovascular disorder. Hence, although the ECG can identify individuals with occult cardiovascular disease, the role and cost-effectiveness of screening of athletes has not been established.

Conclusion

A number of drugs and electrolyte abnormalities may result in prolongation of the QT interval and risk of ventricular arrhythmias. Assessment of the QT interval, corrected for heart rate, should be made routinely with the use of drugs known to prolong the QT interval. The QT interval may also be prolonged as a congenital syndrome associated with risk of sudden death. Long QT syndrome, as with other sudden death syndromes, should be managed in specialized multidisciplinary clinics, including support from specialists in clinical genetics.

Further Reading

Al-Khatib S, LaPointe NM, Kramer JM, Califf RM. What the clinicians should know about the QT interval. *JAMA* 2003; **289**: 2120–7.

Corrado D, Pelliccia A, Heidbuchel H, *et al*; Section of Sports Cardiology, European Association of Cardiovascular Prevention and Rehabilitation; Working Group of Myocardial and Pericardial Disease, European Society of Cardiology. Recommendations for interpretation of 12-lead electrocardiogram in the athlete. *Eur Heart J* 2010; **31**: 243–59.

Heart Rhythm UK Familial Sudden Death Syndromes Statement Development Group. Clinical indications for genetic testing in familial sudden cardiac death syndromes: A HRUK position statement. *Heart* 2008; **94**: 502–7.

Pelliccia A, Di Paolo FM, Quattrini FM, *et al*. Outcomes in athletes with marked ECG repolarization abnormalities. *N Engl J Med* 2008; **358**: 152–61.

SECTION SIX 06

Cardiomyopathy and Pericardial Disease

26	Hypertrophic cardiomyopathy
27	Dilated cardiomyopathy
28	Restrictive cardiomyopathy
29	Pericarditis
30	Pericardial effusion

PROBLEM

26 Hypertrophic cardiomyopathy

Case History

A 24-year-old man was brought into the emergency department following an episode of syncope during a game of football. He has no known history of medical illness and does not use any regular medications. However, on further enquiry he confessed to intermittent light-headedness previously during football games. He also mentioned that his brother died at the age of 23 years, but the cause of death was not clear. On examination, his blood pressure was 118/78 mmHg, with a heart rate of 68 beats/minute. There was a soft systolic ejection murmur. His electrocardiogram (ECG) showed voltage criteria for left ventricular hypertrophy and strain pattern.

What is the likely diagnosis?

How would you manage this case?

Background

How would you manage this case?
This man gives a history of exertional symptoms with a family history of sudden unexplained death. He has an ejection systolic murmur on examination and his resting

ECG is abnormal with ST/T wave changes. These findings suggest an inherited cardiomyopathy, particularly hypertrophic cardiomyopathy (HCM).

HCM is inherited as an autosomal dominant trait caused by mutations of genes encoding for protein components of sarcomere proteins. As the name suggests, HCM is characterized by left ventricular hypertrophy, which is typically, although by no means exclusively, asymmetrical (septum more than lateral wall) and in the absence of other causes of hypertrophy. The family of the patient with HCM should be offered screening and risk assessment. Of note, HCM can present at any age.

The diagnosis of HCM relies on demonstration of left ventricular hypertrophy, usually with a wall thickness cut-off of 15 mm, with or without systolic anterior motion (SAM) of the mitral valve (believed to be due to drag or Venturi effect) and outflow tract gradient (due to SAM or muscular apposition in the mid-left ventricular cavity). However, HCM may also be associated with lesser degrees of hypertrophy (e.g. 13 mm), which may be difficult to differentiate from other causes of left ventricular hypertrophy. For example, differentiating HCM from hypertension-related hypertrophy in the elderly may rely on demonstration of hypertrophy disproportionate to blood pressure elevation if other features associated with HCM such as SAM are absent. Other imaging modalities (e.g. cardiac magnetic resonance imaging) and tissue Doppler imaging have also been used to differentiate HCM from physiological hypertrophy in athletes.

In this case, transthoracic echocardiography was performed, which confirmed asymmetrical left ventricular hypertrophy with a maximal wall thickness of 25 mm (Figure 26.1). Left ventricular ejection fraction was normal. There was SAM of the mitral valve associated with mild posteriorly directed mitral regurgitation and an outflow tract gradient of 35 mmHg at rest. Generally, left ventricular outflow tract obstruction is defined as a gradient of at least 30 mmHg on continuous wave Doppler on echocardiography, either at rest or on provocation. Although an outflow tract gradient is common, particularly on provocation, it is not invariable. Hence, the term hypertrophic cardiomyopathy as opposed to hypertrophic obstructive cardiomyopathy is preferred.

Treatment of patients with HCM should be driven by symptoms and the individual patient's risk of sudden cardiac death (Figure 26.2). Symptoms may include exertional

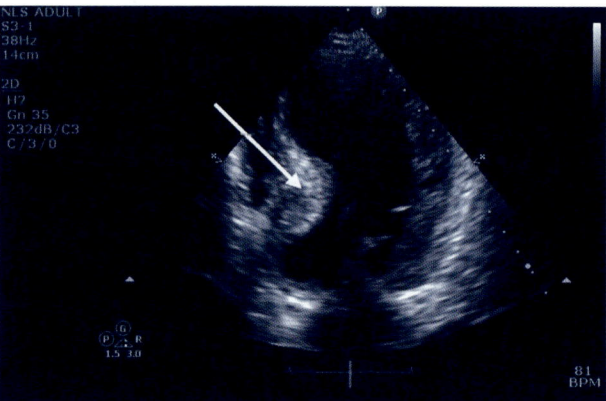

Figure 26.1 A transthoracic echocardiogram demonstrating marked thickening of left ventricular walls with a prominent septal bulge (arrow).

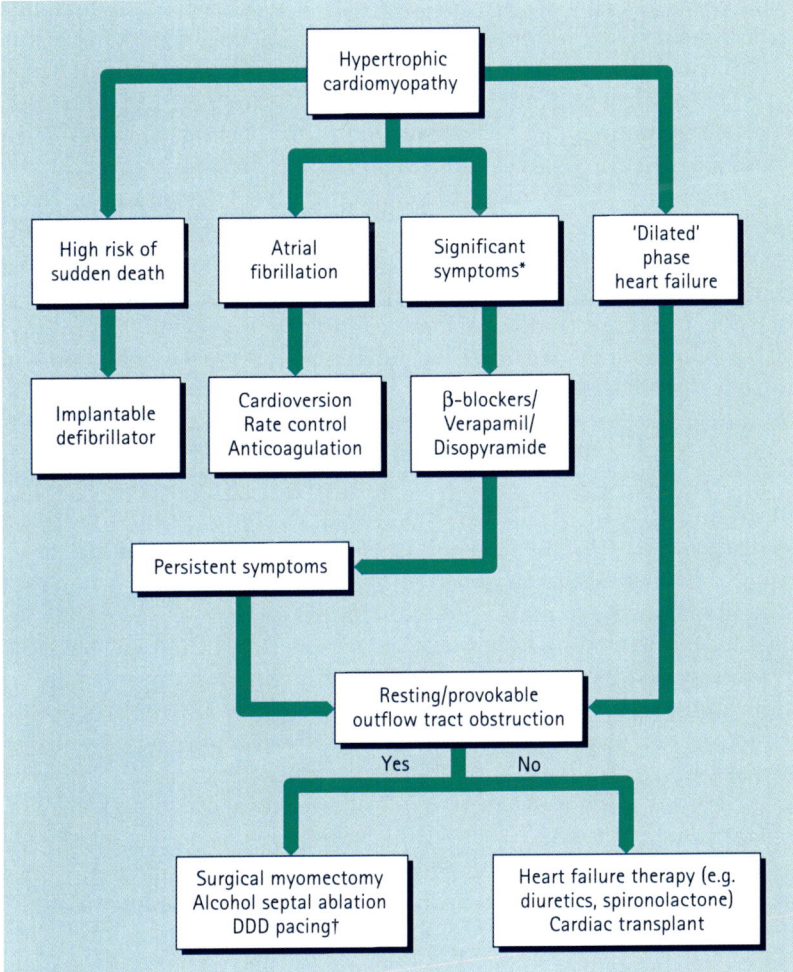

Figure 26.2 Management of hypertrophic cardiomyopathy. *Symptoms may be variable, including chest pain, effort intolerance or pre-syncope. †DDD pacing to pre-excite right ventricular apex/distal septum.

dyspnoea, chest pain (which may be typical or atypical of angina), syncope or presyncope, palpitations (which may be related to ventricular and supraventricular arrhythmias) and stroke. Symptoms of exertional breathlessness may be due to underlying diastolic dysfunction with mitral regurgitation, outflow tract obstruction and, in some cases, left ventricular systolic impairment. Indeed, worsening of symptoms should prompt a search for deterioration in left ventricular systolic function. Syncope and presyncope may be similarly multifactorial in pathophysiology, including arrhythmias, outflow tract obstruction and abnormal vascular response.

β-blockers, typically at high doses are generally considered the first-line treatment for patients with symptomatic HCM. β-blockers may improve diastolic filling by reducing heart rate and may reduce the outflow tract gradient related to exercise. Verapamil is considered the alternative in patients intolerant of β-blockers. Disopyramide has also been used, usually with β-blockers, as disopyramide may accelerate atrioventricular nodal conduction. The anticholinergic side effects of disopyramide (e.g. dry eyes/mouth, constipation and urinary retention) may be reduced by long-acting preparations.

Surgical intervention to relieve outflow tract obstruction may be considered if symptoms are refractory to medical treatment. Surgical myomectomy (the Morrow procedure) is generally regarded as the 'gold standard' in view of its well-documented effects of relieving outflow tract obstruction, reducing mitral regurgitation, improving exercise capacity and reducing frequency of syncope. There are also some (non-randomized) reports of improved survival with surgical myomectomy in severely symptomatic patients. In experienced centres, operative mortality is generally <3%. Despite these benefits, this procedure is not recommended in asymptomatic or mildly symptomatic patients with obstructive HCM.

Percutaneous alcohol septal ablation has been proposed as an alternative to surgical myomectomy. Alcohol septal ablation involves injection of ethanol into one of the septal perforator branches, usually guided by myocardial contrast echocardiography. In effect, this induces an area of myocardial infarction at the desired location at the septum, which relieves outflow tract gradient acutely as a result of infarction and more chronically as a result of remodelling. Although this technique has been shown to reduce outflow tract gradient and symptoms, clinical experience with this technique remains relatively limited (6–8 years follow-up) compared with surgical myomectomy (over 40 years of follow-up). Furthermore, there are concerns about arrhythmias and progressive remodelling associated with myocardial infarctions. Hence, percutaneous alcohol septal ablation is usually reserved for patients unsuitable for surgery. Dual chamber pacing from the right ventricular apex may also have a (small) role in selected patients with HCM.

Sudden death is the most frequent mode of premature death in HCM. The relationship between sudden death in HCM and physical exertion is well publicized. Indeed, HCM is the most common cause of sudden death in young people. Although there appears to be a predilection for younger patients, sudden death associated with HCM has been described in middle-aged and even older patients. A number of risk factors for sudden death in HCM have been identified (Table 26.1). The risk of sudden death increases with the number of risk factors and implantable cardioverter defibrillators (ICDs) are generally indicated in patients with two or more risk factors.

In this case, the patient underwent exercise testing, which demonstrated an abnormal blood pressure response (<25 mmHg rise in systolic blood pressure). Holter (48 hours) did not demonstrate any ventricular arrhythmia. Hence, this patient has three risk factors

Table 26.1 Risk factors for sudden death in hypertrophic cardiomyopathy
1 Maximum wall thickness >30 mm (multiple segments at multiple levels).
2 Systolic blood pressure response measured each minute during maximal upright exercise in patients <40 years (abnormal blood pressure response to exercise = failure to increase by >25 mmHg or fall from peak during continued exercise >15 mmHg).
3 Non-sustained ventricular tachycardia during 48-hour ambulatory ECG monitoring.
4 History of at least one sudden death in a relative <45 years together with a history of syncope.
5 Resting peak instantaneous left ventricular outflow tract gradient >30 mmHg.

(abnormal blood pressure response, resting outflow tract gradient and family history of sudden death with syncope) and he was implanted with an ICD for primary prevention against sudden cardiac death. He was advised against intense physical exertion.

Patients with HCM are also at risk of atrial fibrillation (AF), which occurs in about 20–25% of patients with HCM. The development of AF may be associated with clinical deterioration with worsening of breathlessness, syncope or even ventricular arrhythmias. A rhythm control strategy is generally recommended in view of the association with worsening of heart failure. Amiodarone may be the most effective treatment for maintaining sinus rhythm. In cases of permanent AF, β-blockers and verapamil are usually effective agents for rate control. All patients with either paroxysmal or permanent AF should be considered for anticoagulation in view of the increased risk of thromboembolism.

Finally, some reports suggest that some patients with the diagnosis of HCM may in fact have undiagnosed Anderson–Fabry disease. This is an X-linked recessive lysosomal storage disease that may present with left ventricular hypertrophy, thus confusing the diagnosis. Enzyme replacement has been shown to improve neurological and renal involvement in this condition.

Recent Developments

A recent large registry study evaluated ICD treatment in 50 patients with HCM over an average follow-up of 3.7 years. This study reported about 20% ICD therapy rate (10.6% and 3.6% per year for secondary and primary prevention). Interestingly, the likelihood of appropriate ICD treatment for ventricular arrhythmia was similar in patients with one, two or three risk factors, suggesting that ICD treatment may be indicated in patients with a single risk factor. In another study, myocardial fibrosis identified on cardiac magnetic resonance imaging was found to be associated with an increased frequency of ventricular arrhythmias. Whether cardiac magnetic resonance imaging can improve risk stratification (for sudden cardiac death) remains to be studied.

Conclusion

The clinical presentation and course of HCM is variable. β-blockers (or verapamil) are usually the first-line treatment for patients with symptomatic HCM. Surgical treatment may be considered in patients with refractory symptoms. In view of the risk of sudden death, all patients with HCM should be risk stratified (echocardiography, exercise test and 48-hour Holter) and ICD considered in high-risk patients.

Further Reading

Frenneaux M. Assessing the risk of sudden cardiac death in a patient with hypertrophic cardiomyopathy. *Heart* 2004; **90**: 570–5.

Maron BJ, McKenna WJ, Danielson GK, *et al.* ACC/ESC clinical expert consensus document on hypertrophic cardiomyopathy. *J Am Coll Cardiol* 2003; **42**: 1687–713.

S06 Cardiomyopathy and Pericardial Disease

PROBLEM

27 Dilated cardiomyopathy

Case History

A 45-year-old man presented to the emergency department with worsening of his breathlessness over the past 2 days, which was associated with a persistent cough with small amounts of clear froth, particularly at night. He denied any chest pain or palpitations. He has no history of cardiovascular disease. On admission, he was noted to be in atrial fibrillation with a heart rate of 140 beats/minute. His jugular venous pressure was noticeably elevated with clear evidence of pulmonary congestion. His blood pressure was measured at 110/82 mmHg. There was also pitting oedema to his knees. On further enquiry, he admitted to symptoms of fatigue and breathlessness on exertion over the last 4 weeks. He had also noticed difficulty in putting on his shoes over the last 2 weeks. His father passed away at the age of 72 years following a myocardial infarction but there is no history of heart disease in the family otherwise. He smokes about five cigarettes a day and drinks 10 units of alcohol a week. He denied illicit drug use. He was not aware of his HIV status.

How would you investigate this man?

How would you treat this man?

Background

The findings from the clinical history and examination are consistent with the diagnosis of heart failure. His exertional symptoms over the 4 weeks prior to admission suggest that the heart failure may have been progressing over this period of time with acute deterioration, probably precipitated by the development of atrial fibrillation over the last 2 days. This man was treated with intravenous diuretics and digoxin orally, which resulted in significant symptomatic improvement paralleled by an improvement in ventricular rate. He was also commenced on perindopril (an angiotensin-converting enzyme inhibitor). Following improvement in his pulmonary congestion, he was initiated on bisoprolol (a β-blocker). He was also commenced on anticoagulation therapy.

Investigation of a patient with newly diagnosed heart failure should include electrocardiogram (ECG), renal/liver function tests, creatinine kinase, inflammatory markers (erythrocyte sedimentation rate and C-reactive protein), serum ferritin/iron/transferring and thyroid function test. Non-specific changes (e.g. T-wave inversion, varying degrees of bundle branch block and Q waves) are common on the ECG. Cardiac imaging is crucial in the diagnostic work-up of patients with heart failure. Echocardiography remains the most widely used imaging modality for the assessment of structural heart disease. Coronary angiography may also be considered in some patients, particularly if cardiovascular risk factors are present (Figure 27.1).

More recently, cardiac magnetic resonance imaging has emerged as an effective modality for the assessment of cardiomyopathies. The use of stress protocols and gadolinium enhancement allows comprehensive assessment of cardiac structure, function, ischaemia, and scarring and tissue characterization (Figure 27.2). The use of cardiac magnetic resonance will undoubtedly expand as it becomes more widely available and it may even obviate the need for coronary angiography.

In selected cases, autoantibodies, carnitine, selenium, lactate levels, drug and infection screen (e.g. HIV and hepatitis C), urine for organic acids and skeletal muscle biopsy may be indicated. Viral serology for the diagnosis of viral myocarditis is generally unhelpful (particularly in adults) as the commonly implicated viruses (e.g. coxsackie B and enterovirus) are ubiquitous and antiviral or immunosuppressive/modulatory treatments have not been shown to improve clinical outcomes. Endomyocardial biopsy is not indicated for the routine assessment of cardiomyopathy, but may be considered in some cases when specific conditions are already suspected on clinical grounds and may be confirmed on biopsy (e.g. Loeffler's syndrome, amyloidosis, endocardial fibroelastosis, haemochromatosis and giant cell myocarditis). Giant cell myocarditis has a particularly fulminant course and may require mechanical support/transplantation.

Symptom-limited exercise testing in combination with respiratory gas analysis (cardiopulmonary/metabolic exercise test) is helpful in defining objectively the cause and degree of functional limitation in patients with cardiomyopathy. Oxygen consumption at

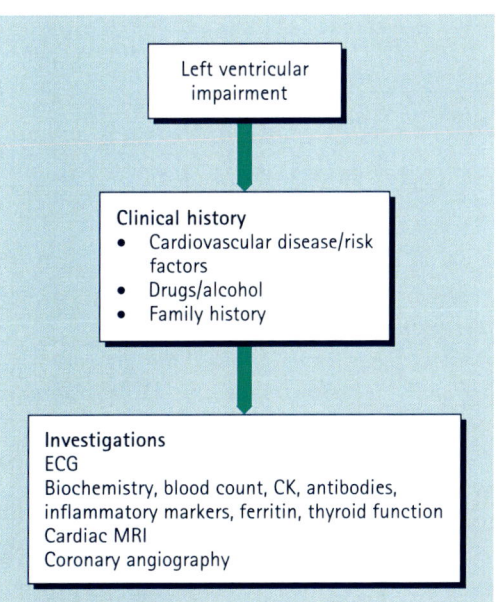

Figure 27.1 Investigation of left ventricle dysfunction. CK, creatine kinase; MRI, magnetic resonance imaging.

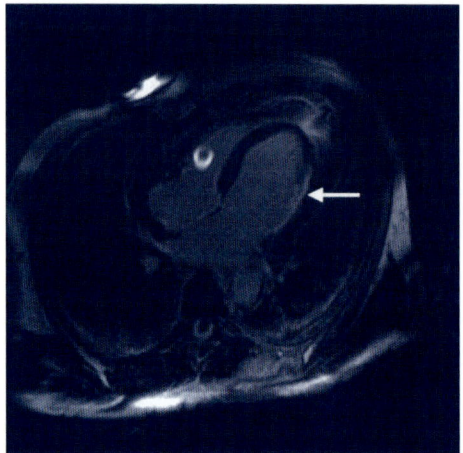

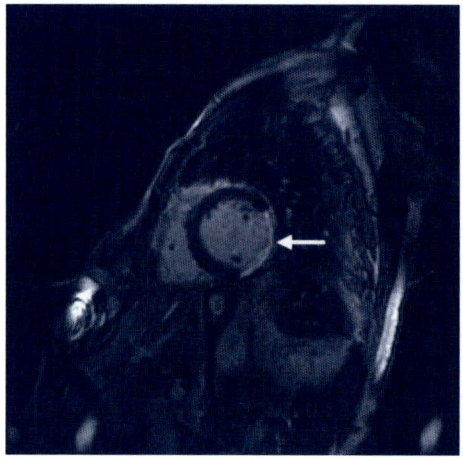

Figure 27.2 Cardiac magnetic resonance imaging with gadolinium enhancement (arrows) of the lateral wall corresponding to infarction of the circumflex artery territory.

peak exercise and ventilatory efficiency are powerful prognostic markers in heart failure and may guide the need for cardiac transplantation.

In this case, transthoracic echocardiography demonstrated a reduced left ventricular ejection fraction of 20–25% and markedly increased left ventricular systolic and diastolic dimensions. There were no regional wall motion abnormalities and no significant valvular abnormalities. His biochemistry and inflammatory markers were normal. He underwent coronary angiography in view of his age and smoking history, which demonstrated no significant flow-limiting stenoses. In the absence of significant occlusive coronary disease, hypertension, alcohol consumption and other causes of left ventricular impairment, this man was diagnosed with 'idiopathic' dilated cardiomyopathy (Table 27.1).

Treatment of patients with dilated cardiomyopathy follows conventional heart failure therapy. There is no specific therapy for most patients with idiopathic dilated cardiomyopathy. A diuretic is the most commonly used treatment for symptoms of fluid over-

Table 27.1 Causes of dilated cardiomyopathy
Ischaemic heart disease
Idiopathic
Familial
Hypertension
Alcohol and toxins (e.g. anthracyclines, trastuzumab and cocaine)
Myocarditis (infective/immune/eosinophilic)
Peripartum
Tachycardia-related
Non-compaction of myocardium
Mitochondrial
Nutritional (e.g. carnitine and thiamine deficiency)*
Anomalous coronary artery or arteriovenous malformation*
Kawasaki disease*
Endocardial fibroelastosis*
*Typically younger patients.

load. This should be combined with an angiotensin-converting enzyme inhibitor or angiotensin II receptor blocker and β-blocker. Spironolactone may be added in patients with persistent moderate–severe symptoms (New York Heart Association [NYHA] III) despite angiotensin-converting enzyme inhibitors and β-blockers. Atrial arrhythmias are common in patients with dilated cardiomyopathy, as in this case. Cardioversion may be attempted but the risk of recurrence is high, particularly in the presence of left atrial dilatation. In patients with persistent/permanent atrial fibrillation, ventricular rate control is important and may be maintained by β-blockers and digoxin if required. Of note, in patients with tachycardia-related cardiomyopathy, left ventricular impairment may recover if rate control is maintained. All patients with atrial fibrillation should be considered for anticoagulation therapy in view of the risk of thromboembolism. The use of anticoagulation therapy in patients with impaired systolic function in sinus rhythm is ongoing.

Patients with dilated cardiomyopathy are also at risk of ventricular arrhythmias. A number of studies have evaluated the use of implantable cardioverter defibrillators as primary prevention against sudden cardiac death in patients with dilated (non-ischaemic) cardiomyopathy. While the overall results favour the use of implantable cardioverter defibrillators, it is clear that the event rates are lower than in patients with ischaemic cardiomyopathy. As such, the absolute benefit is smaller in patients with dilated cardiomyopathy, which renders risk–benefit considerations difficult. The National Institute of Clinical Excellence (NICE) guidelines have excluded patients with dilated cardiomyopathy, although the use of implantable cardioverter defibrillators is recommended by other international guidelines for patients with ejection fractions of <30% with mild–moderate symptoms.

Biventricular pacemakers (cardiac resynchronization therapy) may be considered in patients with severe left ventricular dysfunction, moderate–severe symptoms (NYHA class III or IV) and prolonged QRS duration (>120 ms) despite medical treatment. Patients with significant haemodynamic deterioration may be considered for implantation of ventricular assist devices, which have been shown in some cases to result in significant improvement in left ventricular function. In some cases, this improvement is sustained and has even allowed removal of the device (so-called destination therapy). However, at present, ventricular assist devices are used predominantly as a bridge to transplantation.

Recent Developments

The role of autoimmunity in the pathophysiology of dilated cardiomyopathy continues to be investigated. A recent study suggested autoantibodies directed against β-adrenergic receptors may be relevant and these patients may respond more favourably to β-blocker treatment. Another study found that anti-heart antibodies in relatives of patients with dilated cardiomyopathy may predict the development of cardiomyopathy.

Conclusion

Idiopathic dilated cardiomyopathy is usually a diagnosis by exclusion of other pathology. Cardiac imaging is central to the diagnosis and the use of cardiac magnetic resonance will expand as this technology becomes more accessible. Endomyocardial biopsy has only a limited role in the diagnosis and assessment of dilated cardiomyopathy. Treatment should follow conventional treatment for heart failure. The decision for implantable cardioverter defibrillators for primary prevention against sudden death should be individualized (not recommended by NICE). Patients with progressive deterioration may be considered for cardiac transplantation.

28 Restrictive cardiomyopathy

Case History

A 79-year-old man presented with worsening of peripheral oedema and breathlessness over the last 2 months. This was associated with increasing abdominal swelling. His breathlessness appeared to be worse at nights and he now slept with four pillows. He had also been feeling generally lethargic with loss of appetite over the last 6 months. He believed that he had lost some weight but this was not evident on weighing himself. He denied any chest pain. He has a history of hypertension that is well controlled on amlodipine. He has no known cardiovascular disease. This man is an ex-smoker. On examination, he was breathless at rest. His blood pressure was 100/60 mmHg with an irregular pulse of 110 beats/minute. His jugular venous pressure was clearly elevated with no obvious change with respiration. The apex beat, however, was not displaced. There was evidence of ascites, palpable hepatomegaly and marked peripheral oedema. His electrocardiogram (ECG) confirmed atrial fibrillation with small voltages and non-specific T-wave changes and his chest radiograph demonstrated interstitial oedema consistent with pulmonary congestion and small bilateral pleural effusions but normal cardiac size.

What are the differential diagnoses?

How would you manage this case?

Background

This man has clinical and radiological evidence of fluid overload without clear evidence of cardiomegaly. While normal cardiac size on chest radiograph does not exclude the diagnosis of heart failure, other possible causes of fluid overload must be considered, including renal and liver disease. In this case, routine biochemistry showed elevated alkaline phosphatase with a normal clotting profile, reduced serum albumin and an elevated serum creatinine of 176 μmol/l. Urinary protein excretion rate was measured at about 10 g in 24 hours. Thyroid function test was normal.

Transthoracic echocardiography revealed significant bi-atrial dilatation, and normal ventricular chamber sizes and ejection fraction, but significant hypertrophy of both right and left ventricular (RV and LV) walls. There was also thickening of the atrial septum. Transmitral Doppler indicated a restrictive filling pattern with a short deceleration time of the E wave and reduced A-wave velocity. The inferior vena cava was dilated and the diameter did not change with respiration, which suggests significantly elevated right atrial pressure (consistent with the elevated jugular venous pressure on clinical examination). These echocardiographic findings were noted to be disproportionate to the changes on the ECG (voltages relatively small compared with ventricular hypertrophy).

These echocardiographic findings are consistent with the diagnosis of cardiac amyloidosis and restrictive cardiomyopathy. Restrictive physiology may be demonstrable on echocardiography but will usually require cardiac catheterization. Other features of cardiac amyloidosis include a 'granular sparkling' appearance and thickening of the heart valves, which may be a feature of advanced cardiac amyloidosis. Of note, the 'granular sparkling' pattern, although widely cited, has only low sensitivity and should be applied only to standard echocardiographic imaging (without tissue harmonics). Newer echocardiographic image processing techniques may also reduce the granular appearance. The LV ejection fraction is often normal or nearly normal until late in the disease. As the LV does not dilate, a reduced ejection fraction is associated with a substantially reduced stroke volume and cardiac output. In contrast to LV hypertrophy (e.g. hypertension, aortic stenosis and hypertrophic cardiomyopathy), the thickening of the ventricle in amyloidosis is due to myocardial infiltration, which decreases the ECG voltage (limb leads <5 mm) as the ventricle thickens.

Other causes of restrictive cardiomyopathy are listed in Table 28.1.

Table 28.1 **Causes of restrictive cardiomyopathy**

Infiltrative
 Amyloidosis
 Sarcoidosis
 Gaucher's disease
 Fatty infiltration

Non-infiltrative
 Idiopathic
 Familial
 Hypertrophic cardiomyopathy
 Scleroderma

Storage diseases
 Haemochromatosis
 Fabry's disease
 Glycogen storage disease

Endomyocardial
 Endomyocardial fibrosis
 Hypereosinophilic syndrome
 Carcinoid heart disease
 Drugs/toxins (anthracyclines, ergotamine, methysergide)
 Radiation

How would you manage this case?

As the clinical presentation of restrictive cardiomyopathy may be indistinguishable from constrictive pericarditis, the latter must also be considered in the differential diagnoses. Clinical history may suggest a diagnosis of constriction (e.g. tuberculosis, previous cardiac surgery, radiotherapy) but some causes of constriction may also lead to restrictive cardiomyopathy (e.g. sarcoidosis, amyloidosis). Echocardiography may show some features of cardiac amyloidosis (described above) or thickening of pericardium to suggest the diagnosis. Tissue Doppler imaging for the assessment of long axis function may also be helpful (reduced in restrictive cardiomyopathy). Cardiac catheterization may help distinguish between restriction and constriction (Table 28.2). Of note, unlike restrictive cardiomyopathy, constrictive pericarditis typically results in elevation of venous pressure and right-sided heart failure with minimal pulmonary congestion.

Table 28.2 Haemodynamic findings on cardiac catheterization favouring constrictive pericarditis

Static measurements
  Equalization of end-diastolic pressure (LVEDP-RVEDP >5 mmHg)
  Pulmonary artery systolic pressure >55 mmHg
  Elevated RVEDP (RVEDP/RVSP >1/3)
  Dip and plateau pattern

Dynamic measurements
  Ventricular interdependence (discordant ventricular pressure changes during inspiration)
  Dissociation of intrathoracic and intracardiac pressure (>5 mmHg difference in PCWP-LVEDP between inspiration and expiration)

LVEDP, left ventricular end-diastolic pressure; PCWP, pulmonary capillary wedge pressure; RVEDP, right ventricular end-diastolic pressure; RVSP, right ventricular systolic pressure.

Cardiac amyloidosis may be suggested by typical echocardiographic findings, but the diagnosis of amyloidosis should be confirmed by tissue biopsy that demonstrates apple-green birefringence when stained with Congo red and viewed under a polarizing microscope. The rectal submucosa has been the traditional site for biopsy, which may be complicated by bleeding and perforation. Abdominal fat biopsy is safer and generally more sensitive (about 85%). Endomyocardial biopsy should be performed if the diagnosis is not confirmed by biopsy of other tissue and clinical suspicion is high. Endomyocardial biopsy is generally safe in experienced hands and is almost 100% sensitive due to widespread deposition of amyloid in the heart. Cardiac magnetic resonance imaging (Figure 28.1) with late gadolinium enhancement has also been evaluated recently with a reported sensitivity of about 80% against endomyocardial biopsy as the standard. Where available, radiolabelled serum amyloid P component scintigraphy may

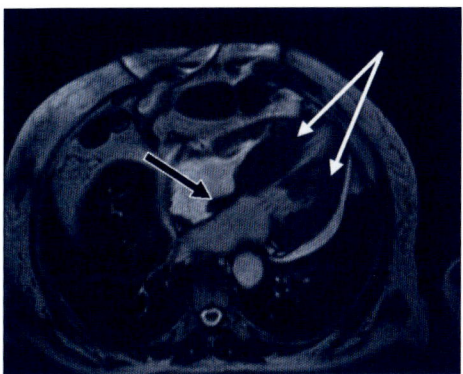

Figure 28.1 Cardiac magnetic resonance imaging of amyloid heart disease. There is gross left ventricular hypertrophy (white arrows) and hypertrophy of the atrial septum (dark arrow).

provide information on the distribution and extent of amyloid deposits throughout the body, and even monitor progress and response to treatment.

Once the diagnosis of amyloidosis is established, the presence of a plasma cell dyscrasia (AL amyloid) should be sought. Echocardiographic features cannot be used to distinguish the different types of amyloidosis. Both serum and urine should be tested for paraprotein. Where available, serum and urine immunofixation should be performed rather than electrophoresis because of greater sensitivity with immunofixation. The recently introduced serum-free light-chain assay is even more sensitive than immunofixation. Bone marrow biopsy is mandatory to assess the percentage of plasma cells and to exclude myeloma and other disorders that can be associated with AL amyloidosis such as Waldenström's macroglobulinaemia.

There are many types of amyloidosis, but significant cardiac involvement is most commonly due to AL amyloid, which is associated with plasma cell dyscrasia and production of amyloid from the clonal immunoglobulin light chain. Cardiac involvement may occur in as many as 50% of patients with AL amyloidosis. Heart failure may be the initial presentation in half of these patients. The majority of patients with AL amyloid have systemic involvement, including the kidneys, liver, dermatological and neurological systems. Hepatomegaly is common and may be a result of congestion from cardiac amyloidosis or amyloid infiltration. Splenomegaly, however, is rare. Renal involvement is common and nephrotic syndrome may exacerbate peripheral oedema. Macroglossia may be found in 10–20% of cases and periorbital purpura is considered pathognomonic of AL amyloidosis. Carpal tunnel syndrome is also common and may precede other manifestations of the disease. Autonomic neuropathy may result in postural hypotension. Indeed, hypertension is unusual and resolution or apparent control of hypertension may be observed. Hence, the diagnosis of cardiac amyloidosis should prompt the search for systemic involvement. The proteinuria in this case was secondary to renal involvement.

Treatment of restrictive cardiomyopathy typically requires diuretic therapy, but excessive diuresis may compromise ventricular filling and further reduce cardiac output. Diuresis may also be difficult in the presence of renal involvement and treatment should be closely monitored. The development of atrial fibrillation (about 25% of patients with cardiac amyloid) may precipitate symptomatic and haemodynamic deterioration due to the loss of atrial contribution and shortened ventricular filling time during rapid ventricular rates. It is therefore important to maintain sinus rhythm (usually with amiodarone). Digoxin should be used with caution (for the purpose of ventricular rate control), particularly in patients with amyloidosis, due to the risk of arrhythmia. All patients with atrial fibrillation should be considered for anticoagulation therapy due to the significant risk of thromboembolism. In some cases, failure of sinus node function or atrioventricular conduction will require permanent pacemakers.

Specific treatment of amyloidosis requires specialist management. Although the overall prognosis remains poor, recent studies suggest that chemotherapy targeting clonal plasma cells that produce the monoclonal immunoglobulin light chains can lead to regression of deposits, preservation of organ function and enhanced survival in patients with AL amyloidosis. High-dose chemotherapy with autologous stem cell rescue (stem cell transplantation) has also been used, but treatment-related mortality may be as high as 25%. Sequential cardiac and stem cell transplantation may also be feasible in younger patients with cardiac amyloidosis without extracardiac involvement. In this case, the patient was not suitable for cardiac transplantation and declined chemotherapy. He passed away 6 months later.

Recent Developments

The distinction between constrictive and restrictive physiology is difficult. Imaging techniques such as computed tomography or magnetic resonance imaging of the heart are widely used but often unhelpful as pericardial thickening is not always present. Direct haemodynamic measurements are usually required.

Static measurements of RV and LV pressures generally lack sensitivity and specificity. Recently, the ratio of RV and LV systolic pressure area (i.e. the area encompassed by the systolic pressure waveform) in inspiration versus expiration – the systolic area index – has been shown to be highly sensitive and specific for discriminating constrictive from restrictive physiology (Figure 28.2). This is based on the concept of ventricular interdependence imposed by constriction (RV and LV filling is dependent on each other as the total cardiac volume is fixed by pericardial constriction). The systolic pressure area typically increases in the RV but decreases in the LV during inspiration (ratio of RV:LV pressure area increase in inspiration), but the converse occurs in expiration. In the absence of ventricular interdependence, RV pressure areas reduce in inspiration and increase in expiration with relatively unchanged LV pressure area (ratio of RV:LV decreases in inspiration but increases in expiration). Hence, the systolic area index in constriction should be higher in constriction than restriction. Indeed, a systolic area of >1.1 is highly sensitive and specific for constriction.

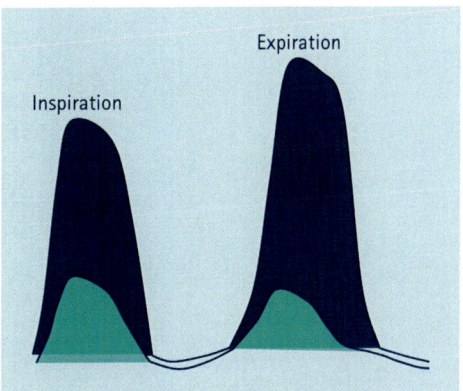

Figure 28.2 Systolic area index and ventricular interdependence. In the setting of constriction, the overall volume is fixed, resulting in interdependence between the right and left ventricles (RV and LV). Increased venous return during inspiration increases RV filling at the expense of LV filling. Hence, during inspiration, the RV pressure increases (the RV systolic area in green increases) but LV pressure decreases (LV systolic area in blue reduces). The converse occurs during expiration.

Conclusion

Restrictive cardiomyopathy often presents with breathlessness, fatigue and fluid overload. Restrictive cardiomyopathy shares many similarities with constriction and differentiating the two conditions can be challenging. Amyloidosis, particularly AL amyloid is one of many causes of restrictive cardiomyopathy. Management of cardiac amyloidosis is difficult and will usually require specialist input as treatment of amyloidosis continues to develop.

Further Reading

Falk RH. Diagnosis and management of the cardiac amyloidoses. *Circulation* 2005; **112**: 2047–60.

Kushwaha SS, Fallon JT, Fuster V. Restrictive cardiomyopathy. *N Engl J Med* 1997; **336**: 267–76.

29 Pericarditis

Case History

A 20-year-old man presented to the emergency department with gradually worsening sharp, central chest pain over the last 24 hours, which radiated to the scapula. He is normally very active and other than a recent flu-like illness, he does not have any significant medical history. He does not take any medications normally and denied any illicit drug use. There is no family history of heart disease. At presentation, he was in obvious discomfort. His temperature was 37.2°C. His breathing was shallow as it hurt to take deep breaths. On auscultation, there appeared to be some added high-pitched sounds in addition to his normal heart sounds. His blood pressure was stable and there were no signs of heart failure. His electrocardiogram (ECG) is shown in Figure 29.1.

What is the likely diagnosis?

How would you investigate this man?

How would you treat this man?

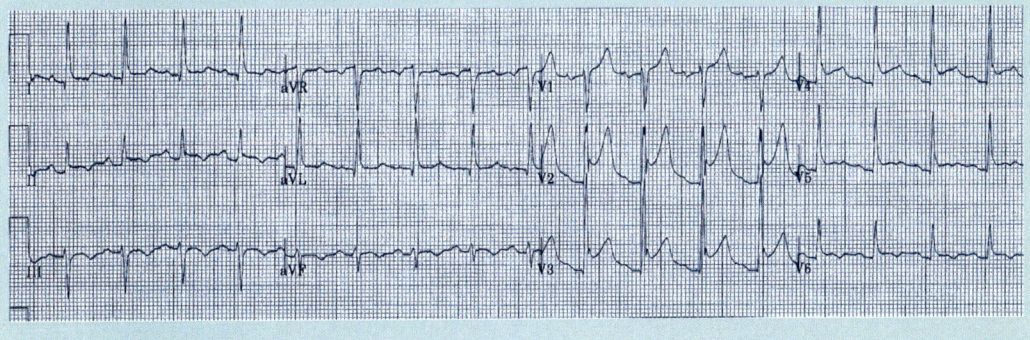

Figure 29.1 Widespread saddle-shaped ST elevation and PR segment depression.

Background

The recent flu-like illness, and sharp and pleuritic chest pain is suggestive of acute pericarditis. On further questioning, he describes his chest pain to be worse lying supine and easier leaning forward, which is consistent with pericarditis. The added heart sounds are likely to be pericardial rubs, which are usually high pitched and scratchy in nature. In some cases, three components of the pericardial rub may be identified: during ventricular systole, diastolic filling and atrial systole (absent in atrial fibrillation). The characteristics of pericardial rub often change even on the same day and the presence of a rub does not exclude possible pericardial effusion. There is often a low-grade fever associated with elevation in circulating leucocytes and inflammatory markers. The causes of pericarditis are listed in Table 29.1. Tuberculous pericarditis is more prevalent in developing countries. In this case, the diagnosis is likely to be acute viral pericarditis.

The ECG may show widespread ST elevation and PR segment depression as in this case (Figure 29.1), which is consistent with acute pericarditis. The pattern of ST elevation does not usually correspond to any specific coronary artery territory and typically spares lead aVR, which may differentiate it from acute myocardial ischaemia. The ECG may be normal in acute pericarditis as it progresses from ST/PR segment changes to normalization of these segments, followed by T-wave inversion and finally normalization of the T waves. It is unusual to find T-wave inversion with persistent ST elevation in acute pericarditis alone, and this finding should prompt a search for possible ischaemia or myocarditis.

Table 29.1 Causes of pericarditis

- Idiopathic
- Infection (viral, bacterial, tuberculous, fungal)
- Uraemic
- Neoplasm
- Acute myocardial infarction (acute or delayed)
- Traumatic (including cardiac surgery)
- Systemic inflammatory disease (e.g. rheumatoid arthritis, systemic lupus erythematosus, Reiter's syndrome)
- Radiation treatment

How would you investigate this man?

Cardiac troponin is frequently, and unnecessarily, requested in patients with chest pain. Troponin elevation is common (up to 50%) in patients with acute idiopathic or viral pericarditis, particularly in young men and in association with ST segment elevation. It is not associated with worse outcomes. The diagnosis of viral pericarditis is difficult. A fourfold rise in antiviral antibodies is sometimes used, but is not diagnostic and in the absence of specific antiviral therapy is unlikely to alter clinical management. The definitive diagnosis requires evaluation of pericardial effusion and/or pericardial/epicardial tissue by polymerase chain reaction or *in situ* hybridization, but this is rarely indicated. In general, when pericarditis develops in a condition known to be associated with pericardial disease (e.g. myocardial infarction, systemic lupus erythaematosus or renal failure), it can usually be assumed that both are related and no additional studies are necessary for the aetiological diagnosis.

Echocardiography may be useful for identifying pericardial effusion (with or without tamponade) and features suggestive of possible myocarditis. Idiopathic or viral pericarditis is usually associated with only small non-haemodynamically significant pericardial effusions. Large effusions should raise the possibility of a neoplastic process, tuberculosis, uraemic pericarditis or myxoedema. Rarely, transoesophageal echocardiogram and other imaging modalities (e.g. magnetic resonance imaging) may be needed to assess loculated pericardial effusions. Myocardial involvement (myopericarditis) may result in impairment of ventricular function, but most cases will normalize and have a benign course. More severe or rapidly progressing heart failure is unusual in pericarditis and should raise the suspicion of a dominant myocarditis. In this case, echocardiogram showed normal left ventricular systolic function with only a small, non-significant rim of pericardial effusion. There was no indication for pericardiocentesis.

How would you treat this man?

Treatment of pericarditis should first be targeted at the cause (Figure 29.2). Renal dialysis, for example, may improve uraemic pericarditis. Non-steroidal anti-inflammatory agents (NSAIDs) are the first-line treatment for acute pericarditis. In the setting of pericarditis associated with acute myocardial infarction, aspirin may be preferable to indomethacin or other NSAIDs due to the effect on myocardial recovery. High-dose aspirin (e.g. 650 mg every 6 hours) should be continued for at least 7 days with tapering of treatment subsequently (recurrence may be reduced by dose tapering based on observational studies). Concomitant use of proton pump inhibitors may be required in some patients to reduce the risk of gastrointestinal bleeding.

Most cases will respond to NSAIDs and are self-limiting. Colchicine may be used in cases refractory to NSAIDs or in recurrent cases. The combination of aspirin–colchicine has been shown to be more effective than aspirin alone in preventing recurrence of pericarditis in patients with first episode (COPE study [Colchicine for Acute Pericarditis]) or recurrent pericarditis (CORE study [Colchicine for Recurrent Pericarditis]). Steroids should only be considered if pericarditis fails to respond to NSAIDs and colchicines, or in

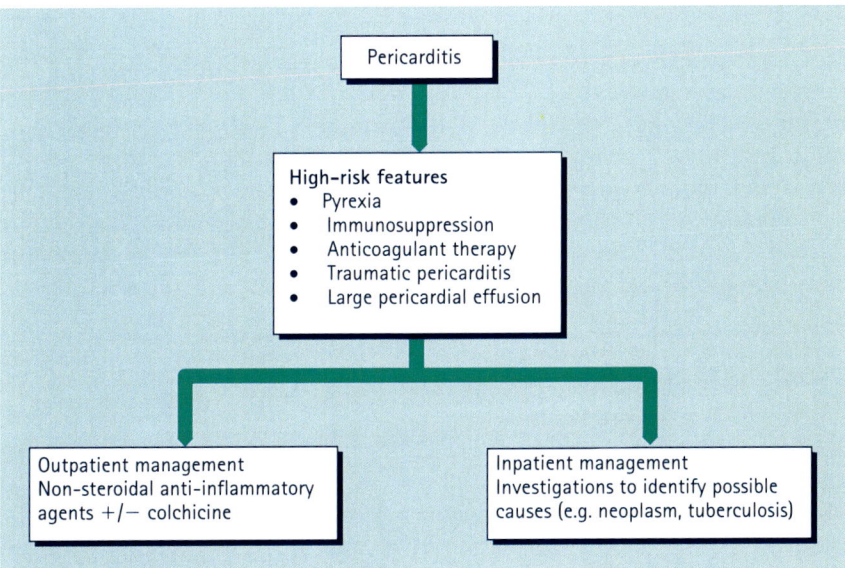

Figure 29.2 High-risk features of pericarditis.

the context of a systemic inflammatory disease, as it is associated with increased recurrence of pericarditis. Potential causes should be carefully sought in these difficult recurrent cases. Intrapericardial steroid treatment and pericardiectomy are rarely required.

Most patients do not require prolonged hospitalization (usually <24–48 hours). Several high-risk features have been identified, which should prompt a detailed investigation for a specific cause (e.g. examination of pericardial fluid) and closer monitoring for potential complications (e.g. pericardial tamponade, constrictive pericarditis or recurrence). Clinical or echocardiographic features associated with poor prognosis are: fever >38°C, subacute onset (several days to weeks), immunosuppression, traumatic pericarditis, oral anticoagulant therapy, severe pericardial effusion (>20 mm or cardiac tamponade) and failure to respond to NSAIDs. Patients without these high-risk features are suitable for outpatient follow-up and treatment. In these low-risk patients, extensive diagnostic evaluation is unlikely to identify a specific cause. In this case, he responded well to aspirin and has no high-risk features. He was discharged after 24 hours for continued outpatient treatment. He has not had a recurrence at 6 months.

Recent Developments

Steroids are rarely indicated in the treatment of pericarditis. When indicated, high doses are generally used. One study compared high-dose steroid (1 mg/kg per day) and low-dose steroid (0.2–0.5 mg/kg per day) for the treatment of pericarditis. This retrospective study of 100 patients reported a higher incidence of side effects and recurrence of pericarditis with high-dose steroids. Hence, if steroid use is considered for the treatment of pericarditis, low doses are preferred.

Conclusion

The diagnosis and assessment of acute pericarditis can usually be made by clinical evaluation and echocardiography. The majority of cases of acute pericarditis are idiopathic or viral in aetiology and most cases will respond to NSAIDs and colchicine. Cardiac troponin is frequently raised and does not indicate a worse prognosis. Fever >38°C, subacute onset, immunosuppression, traumatic pericarditis, oral anticoagulant therapy and severe pericardial effusion are associated with poorer outcome and should prompt a search for possible underlying pathology and closer monitoring for potential complications. Steroids are associated with increased recurrence and should not be used routinely.

Further Reading

Imazio M, Demichelis B, Cecchi E, *et al.* Cardiac troponin I in acute pericarditis. *J Am Coll Cardiol* 2003; **42**: 2144–8.

Little WC, Freeman GL. Pericardial disease. *Circulation* 2006; **113**: 1622–32.

30 Pericardial effusion

Case History

A 48-year-old woman presented with a 3-month history of progressively worsening breathlessness on effort, associated with increasing ankle swelling. She smokes about five cigarettes a day but has no known respiratory or heart disease. On examination, her blood pressure was 120/84 mmHg with a resting heart rate of 102 beats/minute. Her jugular venous pressure was elevated but her chest was clear. Her heart sounds were soft but there were no added sounds. There was pitting oedema to her knees.

How would you investigate this patient?

What are the echocardiographic signs of tamponade?

How would you manage a patient with pericardial effusion?

Background

This patient has clinical features suggestive of heart failure. Investigations should include a 12-lead electrocardiogram (ECG), chest X-ray and echocardiogram. The ECG showed sinus tachycardia with small amplitude but no other abnormalities. The chest X-ray showed a globular enlarged heart but lung fields were clear. The echocardiogram confirmed a 2.5-cm echo-free space consistent with a global pericardial effusion with collapse of the right atrium and right ventricle in diastole (Figure 30.1). Left ventricular function was hyperdynamic. This patient, therefore, has a large pericardial effusion with echocardiographic features suggestive of cardiac tamponade.

In retrospect, the soft heart sounds were consistent with significant pericardial effusion. Further examination of blood pressure revealed a paradoxical pulse (pulsus paradoxus), which refers to a drop in systolic blood pressure of at least 10 mmHg with inspiration. Hence, the astute physician may detect clinical features of pericardial tamponade. (*Note*: pulsus paradoxus can also be found in constrictive pericarditis and acute asthma. To detect pulsus paradoxus, a blood pressure cuff is gradually deflated from suprasystolic blood pressure until the Korotkoff sound is first detected. The patient is then asked to inspire and the Korotkoff sound may disappear as the blood pressure drops below the cuff pressure, and reappear as the cuff pressure is lowered further). The degree of pulsus paradoxus may be associated with the degree of haemodynamic compromise, but it may be absent in patients with left ventricular dysfunction. The jugular venous pulse, although often elevated, may not be evident if cardiac tamponade is associated with intravascular depletion (e.g. post-dialysis in uraemic pericarditis).

Occasionally, the ECG may show changes associated with pericardial effusion, such as

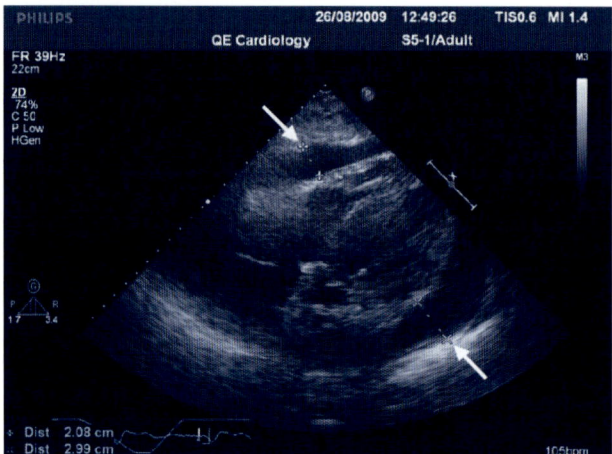

Figure 30.1 Large global pericardial effusion (note measurements, arrows).

globally small voltage amplitude and electrical alternans (Figure 30.2), but these changes lack sensitivity. The cause of the pericardial effusion should be sought (see Table 29.1). Occasionally, the pericardial fluid may be drained for diagnostic purposes, although the diagnostic yield is generally low.

Echocardiogram is extremely valuable for confirming the presence and distribution of pericardial effusion, identifying signs of tamponade, guiding drainage of pericardial fluid and excluding other causes of the patient's condition. Echocardiogram should be performed as soon as possible if cardiac tamponade is suspected. Pericardial effusion appears as an echo-free space but fibrinous strands and thrombus may be present depending on the nature of the effusion. The pericardial effusion may be global (circumferential) or localized. Rarely, small, localized pericardial effusion may cause cardiac tamponade.

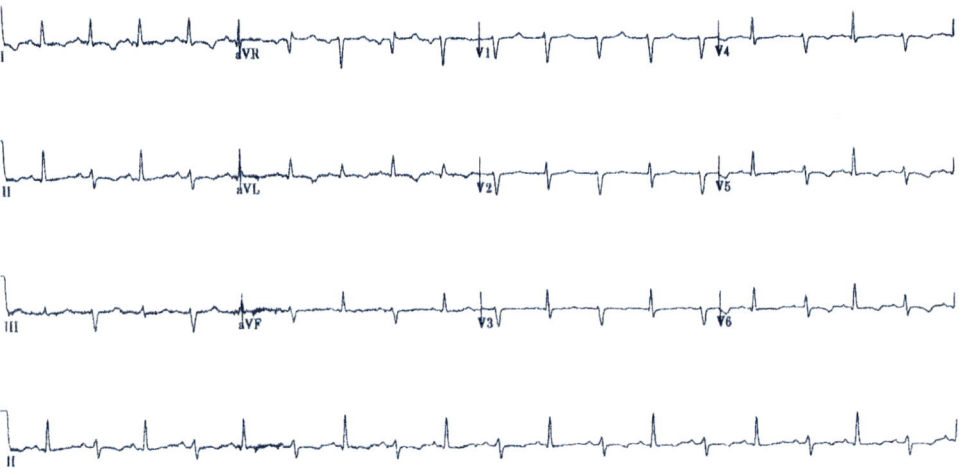

Figure 30.2 QRS alternans. Note alternating QRS axis.

Global pericardial effusion of <1 cm in depth is considered small, moderate if it is 1–2 cm and large if the effusion is >2 cm (generally >700 ml).

Echocardiographic features of cardiac tamponade reflect the haemodynamics and pathophysiology of tamponade. As the right atrium and ventricle are low-pressure structures, they are more likely to be compressed. Hence, right atrial collapse is a sensitive but non-specific sign of cardiac tamponade. Right ventricular collapse, particularly if it lasts for more than a third of the diastole, is more specific for tamponade. As venous pressure increases, the inferior vena cava may be distended and may not show evidence of collapse with inspiration (the inferior vena cava normally diminishes in diameter during inspiration as venous return increases with inspiration).

Cardiac tamponade results in constraint of the pericardial space. As a result, increased filling of the right ventricle must necessarily reduce filling (and therefore output) of the left ventricle. Hence, during inspiration, venous return increases and flow across the tricuspid valve increases (detectable by Doppler echocardiogram), at the expense of left ventricular filling (hence, flow across the mitral valve reduces during inspiration). The converse occurs during expiration. A change in flow velocities of at least 25% is considered significant. This reciprocal respiratory variation in mitral and tricuspid flow velocities is more specific for cardiac tamponade and reflects 'ventricular interdependence'. Indeed, ventricular interdependence is also the pathophysiological basis for pulsus paradoxus. These haemodynamic changes are also seen in constrictive pericarditis and differentiate it from restrictive cardiomyopathy.

Drainage of the pericardial effusion is the treatment for cardiac tamponade. Often, the haemodynamic response to drainage in the setting of acute severe tamponade is almost immediate. Fluid resuscitation may result in transient improvement but continued aggressive administration of intravenous fluid may be detrimental. Inotropes are generally unhelpful as cardiac contractility is not the primary abnormality, and there is usually already significant adrenergic stimulation in response to the reduced cardiac output. Positive pressure ventilation may precipitate haemodynamic collapse.

The management of non-traumatic pericardial effusion without clinical evidence of tamponade is more controversial in the absence of specific randomized studies and variable (and even conflicting) small reports of the risk of progressing to tamponade. Isolated diastolic collapse of the right heart on echocardiogram without evidence of haemodynamic instability (e.g. systolic blood pressure >110 mmHg without pulsus paradoxus) may not require immediate pericardial drain. Pericardial drain is generally recommended for large (>2 cm) pericardial effusions of recent onset (<1 month) with evidence of right heart collapse. It is generally believed that more gradual accumulation of pericardial fluid (e.g. in malignancy) may allow dilatation of the pericardium (more compliant) and is therefore less likely to result in cardiac tamponade. Drainage in these cases may not be necessary (Figure 30.3). However, all these patients require careful regular assessment.

Some pericardial effusions reoccur, particular malignant effusions. These cases may be best served by a pericardial window (into the pleural space) created surgically or even a percutaneous balloon technique.

In this case, the patient underwent a pericardial drain insertion and about 1 litre of blood-stained pericardial fluid was removed. Further investigations revealed advanced metastatic ovarian malignancy. There was reaccumulation of the pericardial fluid (1.5 cm), but not sufficient to cause haemodynamic compromise. She did not undergo further drainage and she passed away 6 months later.

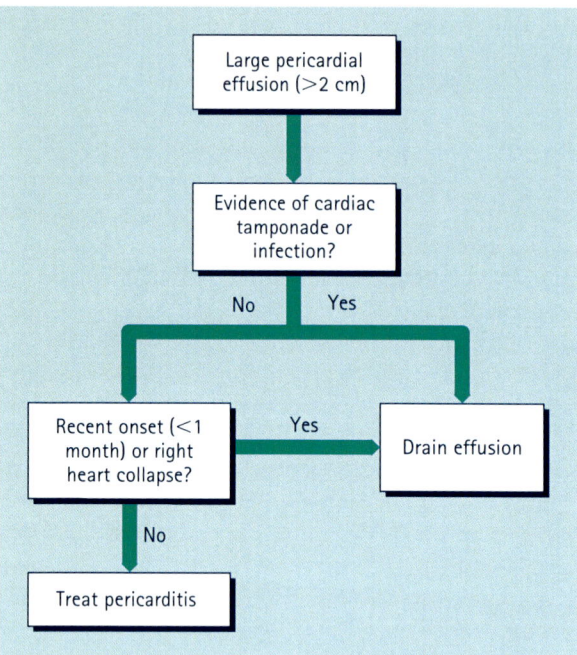

Figure 30.3 Management of pericardial effusion.

Recent Developments

A recent systematic review reported on the sensitivity and specificity of various clinical signs and symptoms for the diagnosis of pericardial tamponade. Almost 90% of patients will have symptoms of dyspnoea, but hypotension has a very poor sensitivity for diagnosing pericardial tamponade. Pulsus paradoxus of >10 mmHg (about 80%), elevated jugular venous pressure (about 75%) and cardiomegaly on chest X-ray (about 90%) are relatively sensitive for the diagnosis of tamponade.

Conclusion

Cardiac tamponade is not an all-or-none phenomenon. It is a haemodynamic continuum, which reflects the interaction between intrapericardial and intracardiac pressures. The effect of a pericardial effusion may range from no haemodynamic compromise to the syndrome of heart failure and in some cases circulatory collapse. Although a large collection is more likely to result in tamponade, this is not invariably so, and even a small loculated pericardial effusion may cause haemodynamic compromise. The diagnosis and assessment of pericardial effusion and cardiac tamponade require a combination of clinical and echocardiographic evaluation, and the decision to drain the effusion should be based on these assessments.

SECTION SEVEN   07

Congenital Heart Disease

31	Ventricular septal defect
32	Atrial septal defect and patent foramen ovale
33	Tetralogy of Fallot
34	Coarctation of aorta
35	Contraception in congenital heart disease

PROBLEM

31 Ventricular septal defect

Case History

A 45-year-old man presented to his doctor for a routine check-up. He is concerned about the risk of heart attack, as his father has recently been treated for angina. He is normally very active and plays tennis twice a week. There is no past medical history of note. There is no family history of heart disease otherwise. On examination, he looked well with a resting heart rate of 64 beats/minute and blood pressure of 120/84 mmHg. However, the doctor has detected a grade 3/6 pansystolic murmur at the lower left sternal edge. There was no evidence of heart failure. The doctor has decided to refer to you for your opinion.

How should this patient be investigated?

What are the different types of defects and what are the indications for closure?

Background

Typical causes of pansystolic murmur include mitral regurgitation, ventricular septal defect (VSD), high pressure tricuspid regurgitation and in some cases of aortopulmonary connections (e.g. patent ductus arteriosus), the presence of elevated pulmonary vascular resistance. As this man is asymptomatic, the latter two are unlikely. A transthoracic echocardiogram is particularly useful for the assessment of possible VSD or mitral regurgitation. The location of the VSD, valvular abnormalities, left ventricular size and function, and pulmonary artery pressure can usually be determined from echocardiography. A transoesophageal echocardiogram may be used in some cases to define the anatomy. In this case, the echocardiogram and magnetic resonance imaging (Figure 31.1) demonstrated a small perimembranous VSD with normal pulmonary artery pressure, left ventricular size and function, and no significant valvular abnormalities. In some cases, right heart catheterization may be performed if the haemodynamic significance of the VSD is in doubt.

Electrocardiographic changes are dependent on the effect of the VSD on the heart. Significant shunting through the VSD may result in biventricular enlargement with large biphasic RS complexes in the mid-precordial leads. Prolongation of the PR interval may be observed in about 10% of patients with VSD and there is a 1–3% risk of progression to complete heart block. However, the electrocardiogram is often unremarkable in patients with small non-haemodynamically significant defects. An increased frequency of ventricular ectopics may also be observed.

What are the different types of defects and what are the indications for closure?

VSDs are the most common cardiac defect, occurring in about 1 in 500 live births and accounting for about 20% of cardiac malformations. This is due to the complexity of the embryological development of the ventricular septum. Generally, the ventricular septum can be divided into a membranous and a muscular section; about 80% of all VSDs occur at the junction between the two and are termed perimembranous VSDs (Figure 31.2). Muscular VSDs (at the muscular septum) are the next most common. The endocardial cushion and outlet septum type VSDs are rare and may be associated with significant valvular abnormalities.

Patients with large VSDs, which allow larger volumes of blood to be shunted (usually from the high-pressure systemic circulation to the low-pressure pulmonary circulation, i.e. left-to-right shunt), usually present early in infancy or childhood with breathlessness,

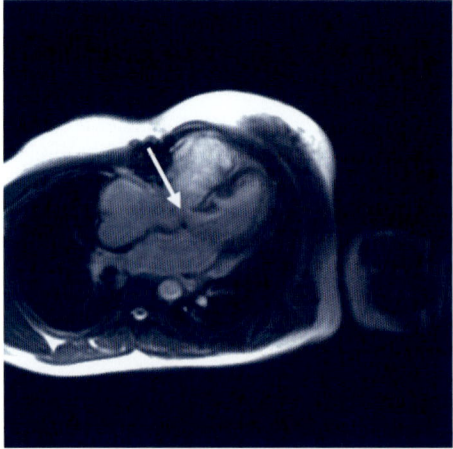

Figure 31.1 Cardiac magnetic resonance imaging demonstrating a perimembranous ventricular septal defect (arrow).

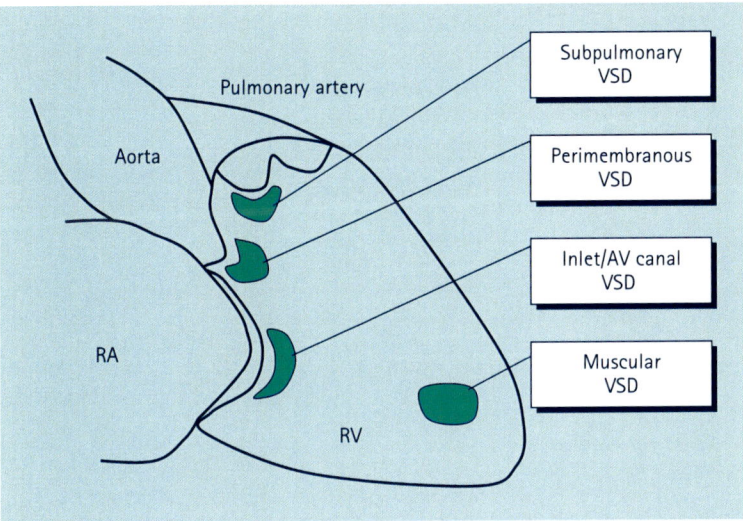

Figure 31.2 In this view, the free walls of the RA and RV are removed, viewing the ventricular septum directly. The presence of perimembranous VSD may compromise support for the aortic valve. AV, atrioventricular; RA, right atrium; RV, right ventricle; VSD, ventricular septal defect.

progressive heart failure and failure to thrive. Recurrent respiratory infection is also common. If they survive without treatment, the shunting of blood into the pulmonary circulation may result in the development of pulmonary hypertension and right heart failure. As the pressure in the pulmonary circulation increases beyond that of the systemic circulation, the shunt may reverse (right to left), resulting in deoxygenation and cyanosis – Eisenmenger's syndrome. Hence, large VSDs are usually closed in infancy to avoid these complications.

Patients with only small VSDs may be asymptomatic and are frequently detected during routine assessment. Some of these small VSDs may close spontaneously. Clinically, significant shunting is unlikely in adults with small VSDs without heart failure or pulmonary hypertension. These VSDs do not need to be closed for treatment of potential left-to-right shunting (Figure 31.3). However, they may be closed for other reasons, such as endocarditis or clinically significant aortic incompetence due to inadequate support of the coronary cusps. Of note, although these small VSDs may not be clinically significant, they often generate a loud pansystolic murmur (Maladie de Roger), as in this case. In contrast, elevation of right ventricular pressure and equalization of pressure with the left ventricle may reduce the pressure gradient and diminish the intensity of the murmur. Hence, greater intensity of the murmur does not indicate greater haemodynamic severity of the VSD.

In rare cases, the VSDs may be of intermediate size, which are large enough to cause symptoms but not enough to cause significant pulmonary hypertension. These patients, although asymptomatic in childhood, may become progressively more symptomatic as left ventricular compliance reduces with age. The reduction in diastolic filling increases left atrial volume and pulmonary venous congestion. These patients, with signs of heart failure, should be considered for VSD closure.

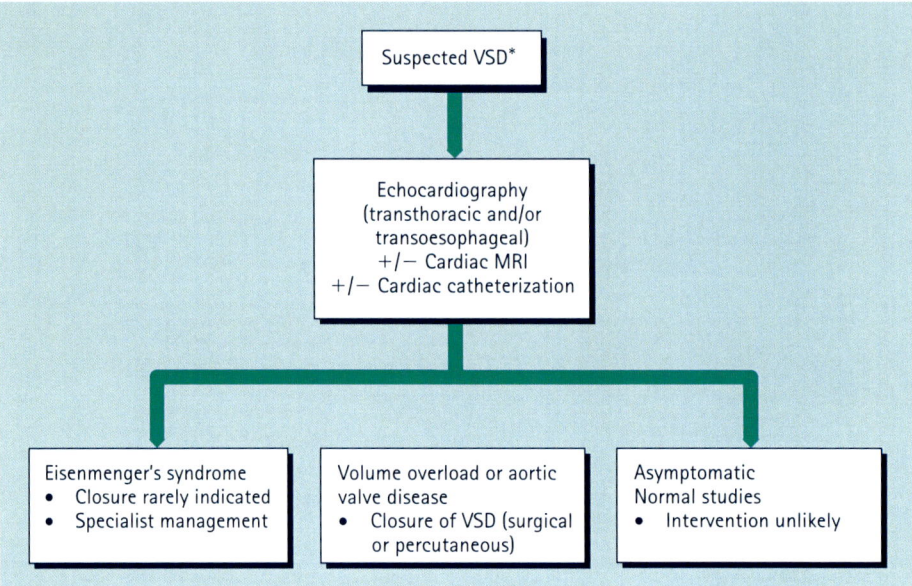

Figure 31.3 Management of ventricular septal defect. MRI, magnetic resonance imaging; VSD, ventricular septal defect. *In an adult patient.

Recent Developments

The last two decades have witnessed considerable progress in percutaneous techniques for VSD closure. Transoesophageal echocardiography is typically used to guide the deployment of these closure devices but intracardiac ultrasound is increasingly used to provide accurate measurements to guide the deployment of the closure device. Although percutaneous closure avoids the risks associated with surgery, the procedure itself carries a 1–2% risk of complete heart block (due to close proximity with the atrioventricular conduction tissue), which may be transient. Damage to the tricuspid valve, with tricuspid stenosis or regurgitation has also been described.

Conclusion

VSDs are the most common cardiac malformation. Small VSDs may generate a loud murmur but are paradoxically less likely to be clinically significant. Small VSDs detected in adults without heart failure or pulmonary hypertension generally do not need to be closed unless there is associated aortic incompetence. Percutaneous closure is associated with a small risk of complete heart block.

Further Reading

Anderson R, Baker E, McCartney F, Rigby M, Shinebourne E, Tynon M. *Paediatric Cardiology*, 2nd Edition. Edinburgh: Churchill Livingstone, 2001.

Julian DG, Cowan JC, McClenachan J. *Cardiology*, 7th Edition. London: WB Saunders, 1998.

Minette MS, Sahn DJ. Ventricular septal defects. *Circulation* 2006; **114**: 2190–7.

PROBLEM

32 Atrial septal defect and patent foramen ovale

Case History

A 17-year-old woman presented to her general practitioner with increasing fatigue and breathlessness on exertion over the last 6 months. She denied any cough or haemoptysis, or any chest pain or palpitations. She has no history of rheumatic fever, and indeed her past medical history was unremarkable. On general examination, she was of average height, but noted to be slim. There was no evidence of pallor, cyanosis or clubbing. She had a soft ejection systolic murmur over the upper left sternal edge. Her heart sounds were otherwise normal. Her chest was clear. Her doctor was concerned about her symptoms and the murmur, and referred her for your opinion.

How would you investigate this patient?

What are the different types of atrial septal defect?

How can atrial septal defects present in an adult?

What are the clinical signs of atrial septal defects?

What are the indications for closure of atrial septal defects?

Background

Ejection systolic murmurs are common in young individuals and, in many cases, may simply reflect physiological flow murmur. However, murmurs should be investigated in a symptomatic patient, as in this case. Transthoracic echocardiogram is a useful investigation in cases such as this to identify any valvular and structural heart disease, and to assess the haemodynamic consequences of these abnormalities (e.g. pulmonary artery pressure). In this case, a transthoracic echocardiogram demonstrated a secundum atrial septal defect (ASD) with mildly dilated right atrium and ventricle. There was left-to-right shunting on Doppler but the pulmonary artery pressure was estimated to be normal. Of note, signal dropout due to imaging artefact in the apical four-chamber view in the region of the atrial septum is frequently seen and should not be confused with an ASD. In some cases, injection of bubble contrast may be required to visualize shunting through an ASD.

An electrocardiogram was performed and this demonstrated an incomplete right bundle branch block and deviation of the frontal plane axis to the right. These findings are consistent with a secundum ASD.

What are the different types of atrial septal defect?

ASDs (abnormal inter-atrial communication) are common and can present at any age. ASDs can be classified into secundum ASD, primum ASD and sinus venosus defects (Figure 32.1). Secundum ASDs involve the foramen ovale and surrounding atrial septum and account for 80% of ASDs. ASDs are particularly common in patients with Down syndrome (particularly atrioventricular septal defects) and DiGeorge syndrome (primum ASD). Primum ASDs and sinus venosus defects may be associated with complex atrioventricular valvular abnormalities and anomalous pulmonary venous drainage respectively.

How can atrial septal defects present in an adult?

Many adults with ASDs may be asymptomatic, although the majority will develop symptoms at some point. Exertional dyspnoea with fatigue is the most common presentation. Closure of ASDs has been shown to improve exercise tolerance. Some patients with ASDs may present with atrial arrhythmia, particularly in older patients. There is an association between ASDs and pulmonary hypertension, although overt pulmonary hypertension is uncommon in adults with ASDs. Rarely, patients may also present with paradoxical

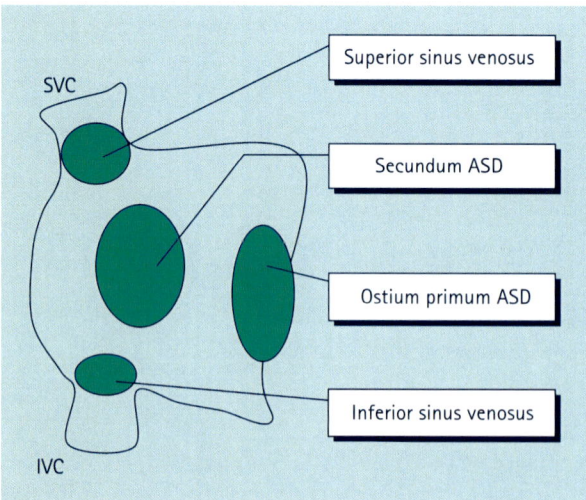

Figure 32.1 Typical location of the different defects is shown in this view of the atrial septum. Primum ASDs are often associated with atrioventricular valvular defects. ASD, atrial septal defect; IVC, inferior vena cava; SVC, superior vena cava.

emboli (embolization from the venous system across the ASD to the arterial system), which may result in stroke and systemic thromboembolism. Primum ASDs usually present at an earlier age due to concomitant valvular defects.

What are the clinical signs of atrial septal defects?

Some patients with ASDs may not have significant signs on clinical examination, even in the presence of haemodynamically significant defects. However, careful examination may reveal a wide and fixed splitting of the second heart sound due to equalization of pressure between the left and right atria throughout the respiratory cycle, which is regarded as the hallmark of an ASD.

An ejection systolic murmur, loudest at the upper left sternal edge, is usually audible and may reflect the increased blood flow through the pulmonary outflow tract. A diastolic rumble at the left sternal edge may represent significant left-to-right shunting and increased flow across the tricuspid valve, creating a 'relative' tricuspid stenosis. A pansystolic murmur may suggest the presence of significant atrioventricular valve defects associated with primum ASDs. Right ventricular lift and a loud second heart sound may reflect pulmonary hypertension. In some cases, cyanosis may only present on exercise (pink at rest) due to pulmonary hypertension on exercise.

The electrocardiogram in over 90% of patients demonstrates a partial or complete right bundle branch block pattern. The precise reason for this is unclear but may relate to selective hypertrophy of the basal portion of the right ventricle, or stretching of the peripheral conduction fibres. The QRS axis in the frontal plane is typically rightward in secundum ASD, particularly in the presence of pulmonary hypertension. Primum ASDs are usually associated with a leftward QRS axis. First-degree heart block suggests primum ASDs, although it may also occur in older patients with secundum ASDs. Atrial arrhythmia (e.g. atrial fibrillation or flutter) may also occur.

Transthoracic echocardiography is a useful first-line investigation as shown in this case (Figure 32.2). Most echocardiographic assessments are performed at rest, and may not identify increases in pulmonary artery pressure on exercise. Exercise studies should be considered in some patients. Although transthoracic echocardiogram can determine the size, location and degree of shunting in experienced hands, transoesophageal echocardiogram is often required to confirm the diagnosis, and determine the size, location and pulmonary venous return (there may be associated anomalous pulmonary venous drainage, particularly in sinus venosus defects). The findings on transoesophageal echocardiography may also guide closure of the ASD.

Cardiac magnetic resonance imaging is widely used as it allows quantification of the shunt, clear assessment of right atrial and ventricular size, and identification of other associated congenital heart defects. Finally, cardiac catheterization may be used to quantify the degree of shunting.

What are the indications for closure of atrial septal defects?

Generally accepted indications for closure of ASDs are:

- haemodynamically significant ASD (generally at least 10 mm in size and pulmonary to systemic flow ratio of at least 1.5 : 1);
- patients with evidence of right ventricular dilatation; and
- patients with a history of systemic thromboembolism.

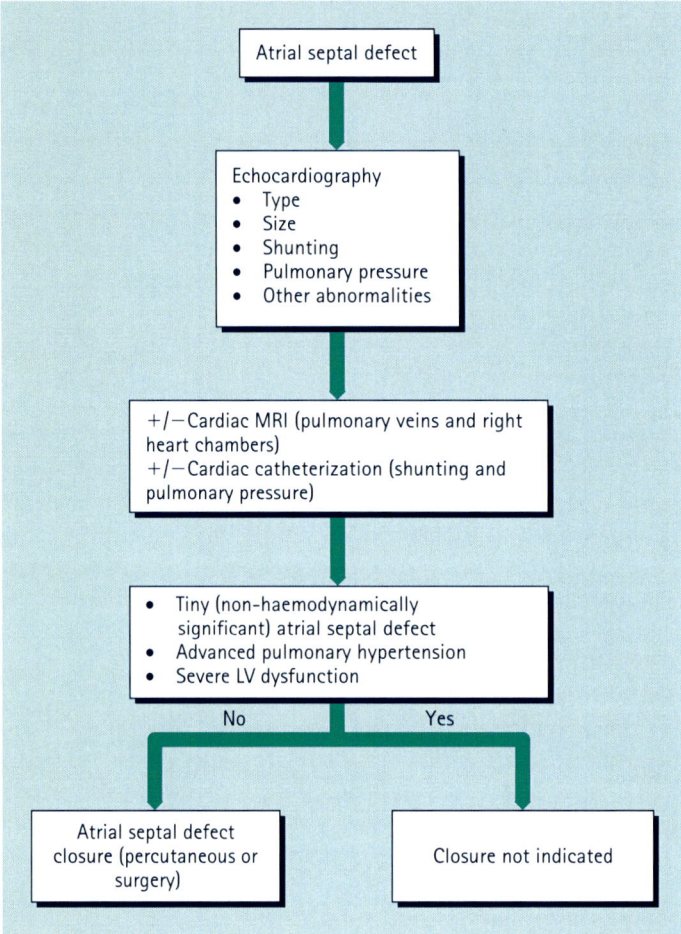

Figure 32.2 Management of atrial septal defect. LV, left ventricular; MRI, magnetic resonance imaging.

Patients with small ASDs and minimal evidence of shunting should be followed up as the degree of shunting may increase as left ventricular compliance increases with ageing. Closure is not recommended in the presence of significant pulmonary hypertension or severe left ventricular dysfunction.

In the setting of suitable anatomy (size of defect, the rim surrounding the defect and proximity of valves), secundum ASDs are now usually closed percutaneously with transoesophageal echocardiographic guidance. Primum ASDs and sinus venosus defects are more complex and typically require surgical closure. Percutaneous device closure (Figure 32.3) is generally safe with <1% risk of major complications (e.g. cardiac perforation and device embolization). Closure of ASDs improves exercise capacity and may prevent systemic thromboembolism and the development of pulmonary hypertension. Long-term complications, even after closure of ASD, may include atrial tachyarrhythmia, brady-arrhythmia (sinus node disease), pulmonary hypertension and right heart failure (risk related to age of ASD closure), device migration and systemic thromboembolism.

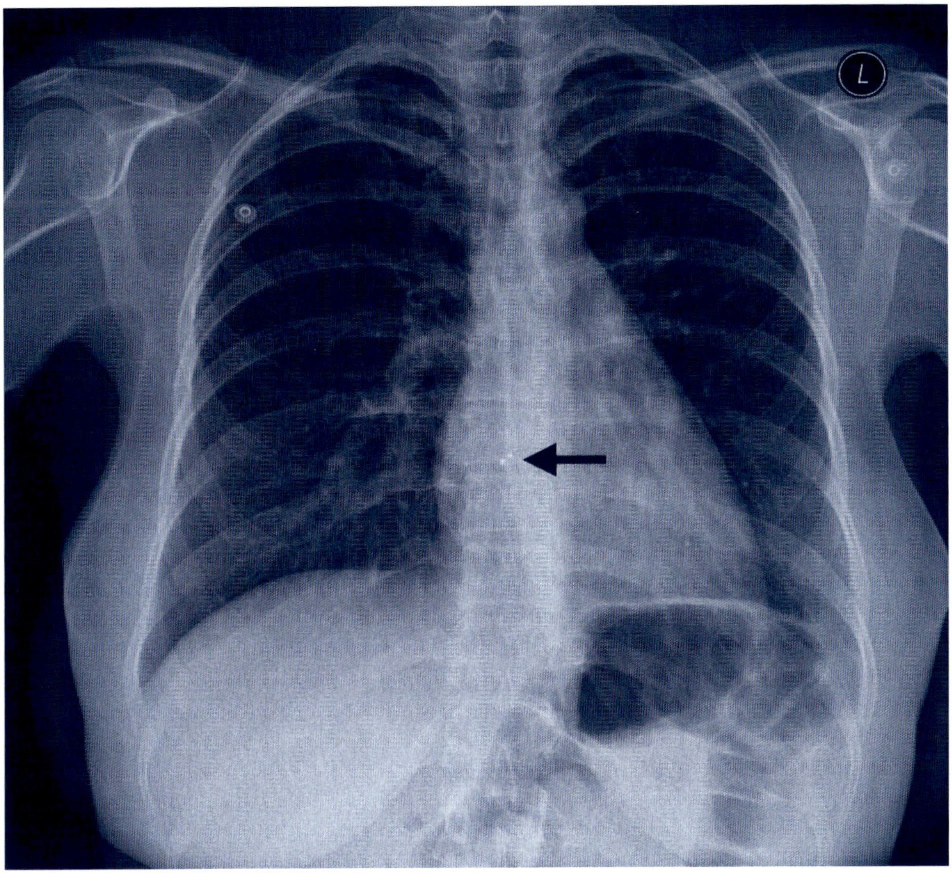

Figure 32.3 Closure device for secundum ASD *in situ* (arrow).

Recent Developments

 Patent foramen ovale (PFO) represents a failure of fusion between the septum primum and secundum, which allows a persistent communication between the right and left atria. The association between PFO and stroke, particularly the so-called cryptogenic stroke is well supported by epidemiological studies. This is generally believed to be due to embolization from the venous circulation across the PFO (right-to-left shunting) to the cerebral circulation, although thromboembolism within the PFO itself is also possible. Indirect comparisons between different studies suggest that closure of the PFO, most commonly by percutaneous techniques, may reduce the risk of recurrent stroke, but direct comparisons in randomized trials are still ongoing.

A randomized, sham-controlled trial of PFO closure has been reported recently. The MIST trial (Migraine Intervention with STARFlex Technology) was performed because of reported associations between migraine and PFO, and small studies suggesting that PFO closure may improve migraine symptoms. There was no significant difference in the primary endpoint of migraine cessation or indeed the various secondary endpoints of

Conclusion

ASDs can present at any age, typically with exertional dyspnoea and fatigue. Secundum ASDs are the most common defects. Complications of ASDs include atrial arrhythmia, systemic thromboembolism and pulmonary hypertension. Closure should be considered in haemodynamically significant ASDs in the absence of significant pulmonary hypertension of severe left ventricular dysfunction. Percutaneous device closure is generally safe and may be suitable for the majority of secundum ASDs.

Further Reading

Webb G, Gatzoulis MA. Atrial septal defects in adults: recent progress and overview. *Circulation* 2006; **114**: 1645–53.

PROBLEM

33 Tetralogy of Fallot

Case History

A 25-year-old woman was admitted to hospital with 4-month history of progressive shortness of breath and abdominal distension. In the past week, she had only been able to mobilize short distances. She had also had some difficulty in fastening her shoes because of ankle swelling. She had no cough or chest pain, but did report occasional palpitations. Her only past medical history of note was a surgical operation for tetralogy of Fallot in childhood. On examination, her blood was pressure was 98/62 mmHg. She was not breathless at rest, but had raised jugular venous pressure with prominent V waves. She had prominent precordial pulsations with moderate ascites and 4 cm hepatomegaly. Cardiac auscultation revealed normal first and second heart sounds and a soft long diastolic murmur over the pulmonary area.

What further investigations would you recommend?

What are the features of tetralogy of Fallot?

What are the late complications of surgical treatment?

Background

 Her chest X-ray shows cardiomegaly with an increased cardiothoracic ratio and increased pulmonary vascular markings, and her electrocardiogram (ECG) shows sinus rhythm with right ventricular hypertrophy and a right heart strain pattern. Hence, the clinical, electrocardiographic and radiological findings are consistent with right heart failure. The prominent V waves of her jugular venous pulse suggest significant tricuspid regurgitation. She was treated with intravenous diuretics with significant improvement in her symptoms.

What further investigations would you recommend?

Transthoracic echocardiogram is usually performed for the assessment of cardiac structure and function, and to quantify the degree of valvular dysfunction. However, previous surgical intervention and distortion of anatomy typically limits transthoracic echocardiographic imaging in these patients (poor images). In contrast, cardiac magnetic resonance imaging may be extremely useful for the assessment of ventricular and valvular function in these patients. Indeed, cardiac magnetic resonance imaging is regarded as the gold standard for the assessment of these patients with complex congenital heart disease. In this case, transthoracic echocardiogram demonstrated severe pulmonary and tricuspid regurgitation with a dilated right ventricle. Right ventricular systolic function was normal. These findings were confirmed on cardiac magnetic resonance imaging.

What are the features of tetralogy of Fallot?

Tetralogy of Fallot is a congenital cyanotic heart disease. The four distinct features, as described by Fallot in 1888, are:

1. Right ventricular outflow tract obstruction (infundibular/pulmonary stenosis).
2. A ventricular septal defect (VSD).
3. Overriding of the aorta over the VSD.
4. Right ventricular hypertrophy.

An atrial septal defect may occur in about 5% of cases (called pentalogy of Fallot). Abnormal development of the pulmonary infundibulum appears to be the primary developmental abnormality with secondary right ventricular hypertrophy and displacement of the aorta. This is the most common cyanotic heart defect that survives to adulthood (Figure 33.1).

Patients with tetralogy of Fallot are cyanotic in view of right-to-left shunt across the VSD, as the right ventricular pressure exceeds that of the left ventricle in the presence of anatomical obstruction to the right ventricular outflow tract (infundibular stenosis). The degree of cyanosis is related to the degree of right ventricular outflow tract obstruction. Obstruction to the pulmonary arterial flow is usually at both the right ventricular infundibulum (subpulmonary area) and at the pulmonary valve. Rarely the pulmonary valve could be absent (pulmonary atresia with VSD, an extreme form of tetralogy of Fallot).

Classical clinical features associated with tetralogy of Fallot, such as severe central cyanosis and finger clubbing, may occur in late infancy or childhood if left unrepaired. By adulthood, patients with unrepaired tetralogy of Fallot are typically cyanotic, polycythaemic, profoundly intolerant of exertion and at risk of potentially catastrophic complications such as arterial thromboembolism, cerebral abscess and haemoptysis. As

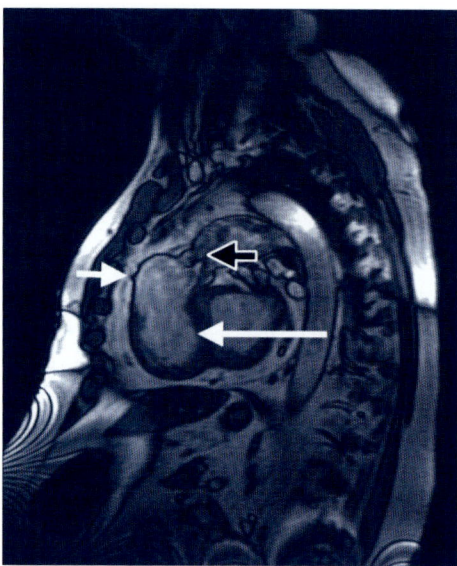

Figure 33.1 A cardiac magnetic resonance imaging of a patient with previous surgical repair of infundibular pulmonary stenosis and ventricular septal defect closure. This magnetic resonance imaging demonstrates dilatation of the right ventricular outflow tract (short white arrow), pulmonary stenosis (note, turbulent flow; short dark arrow) and right ventricular hypertrophy and dilatation (long white arrow).

surgical repair is now performed typically in infancy, these complications are now uncommon.

What are the late complications of surgical treatment?

Early surgical intervention in the 1950s and 1960s were largely palliative and involved shunts to bypass the right ventricular outflow tract obstruction. These included the Blalock–Taussig shunt (subclavian artery to pulmonary artery, which diminishes the radial pulse), the Waterston shunt (ascending aorta to right pulmonary artery) and the Potts shunt (descending aorta to left pulmonary artery). These patients will remain cyanotic and may suffer the same complications later in life as in their unrepaired counterparts. Contemporary surgical repair of tetralogy of Fallot usually involves total surgical correction to separate the pulmonary and systemic blood flow. This typically includes patch closure of the VSD (angled patch to direct blood flow to the aorta) and dilatation of the right ventricular outflow tract, usually with subvalvular muscle resection, pulmonary valvotomy and the placement of a transannular patch.

Late complications following surgical correction of tetralogy of Fallot are seen with increasing frequency as more patients survive into adulthood. Patients presenting with increasing exercise intolerance and heart failure, as in this case, should be investigated for possible residual shunts, residual outflow obstruction, valvular incompetence (particularly pulmonary valve due to previous surgical manipulation) and ventricular contractile dysfunction. Indeed, exercise intolerance and right heart failure is often a cumulative effect of pulmonary regurgitation, consequent right ventricular dilatation and dysfunction, and secondary tricuspid regurgitation (due to annular dilatation), which compounds the right ventricular overload. Patients with pulmonary regurgitation may remain asymptomatic for many years. Pulmonary valve replacement (with tricuspid valve repair) may produce a favourable improvement in symptoms and exercise tolerance, particularly if right ventricular function is preserved. This patient underwent a successful pulmonary valve replacement with tricuspid valve repair.

Patients with repaired tetralogy of Fallot are also at risk of cardiac arrhythmias in adult life. Long-term mortality from sudden cardiac death is about 3–6%. Ventricular ectopics, ventricular tachycardia, sinus node dysfunction and intra-atrial re-entrant tachycardia are also recognized in patients with repaired tetralogy of Fallot. In this case, the presence of palpitations raises the possibility of intermittent tachyarrhythmias and ambulatory monitoring should be considered.

All patients remain at risk of infective endocarditis and should therefore be offered antibiotic prophylaxis prior to dental and relevant surgical procedures at risk of significant bacteraemia.

Recent Developments

Percutaneous techniques are currently being evaluated for the treatment of complications of tetralogy of Fallot. Pulmonary stenosis has been treated with balloon angioplasty. The use of cutting balloons, covered stents and percutaneous pulmonary valves has also been described recently.

Conclusion

Patients with repaired tetralogy of Fallot remain at risk of complications and require regular follow-up. This case highlights the potential risk of right heart failure from pulmonary regurgitation, which may respond well to valve replacement. Other potential complications in patients with repaired tetralogy of Fallot include residual obstruction, residual shunt and ventricular dysfunction. Cardiac magnetic resonance imaging has proven to be extremely valuable in the assessment of cardiac and valvular function in these patients.

Further Reading

Andersen RH, Weinberg PM. The clinical anatomy of tetralogy of Fallot. *Cardiol Young* 2005; **15**(Suppl. 1): 38–47.

Bashore TM. Adult congenital heart disease: right ventricular outflow tract lesions. *Circulation* 2007; **115**: 1933–47.

34 Coarctation of aorta

Case History

A 22-year-old man was referred to the clinic with general fatigue and a recent diagnosis of hypertension. He has no known previous medical history and does not take any regular medications. He denied illicit drug use. On examination, the blood pressure in his right arm was 180/100 mmHg with a resting heart rate of 72 beats/minute. There was an ejection systolic murmur at the left parasternal area on auscultation.

What are the causes of hypertension in the young?

What further investigations will you undertake?

What are the abnormalities associated with coarctation of the aorta?

What are the clinical presentations and the complications associated with coarctation of the aorta?

Background

Conventionally, the causes of hypertension have been divided into either primary 'essential' or secondary hypertension.

Secondary hypertension
- Renal hypertension (renovascular disease)
- Endocrine causes (e.g. phaeochromocytoma, Conn's syndrome, etc.)
- Coarctation of the aorta.

Essential hypertension
Although essential hypertension is occurring in younger patients with increasing frequency, hypertension in this young patient should prompt investigation for secondary causes of raised blood pressure. With this in mind and on further examination, he was noted to have reduced pulsation in his lower limbs compared with his brachial artery with a suggestion of radio-femoral delay. In addition to the ejection systolic murmur, he had a systolic murmur over his left upper back. These clinical findings are consistent with coarctation of the aorta.

What further investigations will you undertake?

This patient had an electrocardiogram, which demonstrated a pattern consistent with left ventricular hypertrophy. Chest X-ray may demonstrate characteristic notching of the undersurface of the ribs, which is related to arterial collateralization to bypass the coarctation. Cardiomegaly may be seen in some cases.

An echocardiogram is useful for the assessment of the severity of the coarctation and to identify other associated structural heart abnormalities. In this case, the echocardiogram showed a thickened bicuspid aortic valve with only a mild gradient across the valve. The proximal aorta was normal in size and continuous wave Doppler showed a gradient of about 24 mmHg in the distal aorta (suprasternal view). In some cases, the characteristic tapering of Doppler signal into diastole may be seen, which suggests significant coarctation. There was no ventricular septal defect. Of note, the pressure gradient across the coarctation may be underestimated by the development of collaterals.

Computed tomography and magnetic resonance imaging provide excellent non-invasive assessment of a patient with coarctation of the aorta (Figure 34.1 – see inside back cover). Imaging can be orientated in any plane, which allows both direct visualization of the site of coarctation and accurate measurement of flow in the descending aorta using velocity mapping, which is possible with magnetic resonance imaging.

What are the abnormalities associated with coarctation of the aorta?

Coarctation of the aorta occurs in about 7% of patients with congenital heart disease. Although it usually presents as a discrete stenosis in the region of the ligamentum arteriosum, more diffuse forms of the disease with variable stenosis of the aortic arch are well described. The stenosis usually occurs distal to the left subclavian artery, which gives rise to the characteristic difference in pulse amplitude and timing between the brachial and femoral arteries (blood pressure measured at the popliteal artery is usually about 10 mmHg higher than the brachial artery). However, the origin of the left subclavian artery may be affected occasionally. The aorta distal to the stenosis is often aneurysmal.

Coarctation of the aorta is associated with a bicuspid aortic valve in up to 40% of cases. There is also an association with intracranial aneurysms, usually in the circle of Willis in about 10% of patients. Less common associations include ventricular septal defects and mitral valve abnormalities. Coarctation of the aorta is more common in patients with Turner's syndrome.

What are the clinical presentations and the complications associated with coarctation of the aorta?

Coarctation of the aorta may present either in the neonatal period (neonatal/infantile type) or later in childhood or adult life (adult type). Neonatal coarctation is often severe in the degree of arch narrowing and often associated with hypoplasia of the aortic arch, which often results in heart failure in infancy. The adult type is often less severe and may escape detection in the neonatal period. Uncomplicated coarctation beyond infancy is often asymptomatic and diagnosed incidentally during the assessment of hypertension and heart murmur. Some adolescents with coarctation may complain about weakness or pain (or both) in legs after exercise.

Long-term complications of coarctation of the aorta include heart failure, the risk of endocarditis, aortic rupture and intracranial haemorrhage due to rupture of associated cerebral artery aneurysms. The risk of heart failure and cardiovascular disease (e.g. stroke and atherosclerosis) is partly related to arterial hypertension, which generally persists even with surgical repair of the coarctation. The associated bicuspid aortic valve may degenerate with time and develop aortic stenosis or regurgitation.

The surgical treatment of coarctation of the aorta and its complications

Surgical treatment of coarctation of the aorta usually includes excision of the area of stenosis with end-to-end anastamosis (with or without an interposed tubular Dacron graft). Other techniques may include the use of prosthetic overlay grafts and patch aortoplasty. Long-term complications of surgical repair include aneurysm formation and recurrent coarctation. All patients with coarctation of the aorta should continue to be followed-up in view of these complications and regular imaging may be required.

Recent Developments

Recent reports on percutaneous balloon aortoplasty, with or without stenting, appear promising (arrows in Figure 34.2 – see inside back cover), and may be suitable for discrete stenosis or patients with recurrent coarctation. Aneurysm formation and the need for repeat intervention (reduced by stenting) are the main limitations of balloon angioplasty compared with surgery.

Conclusion

Coarctation of the aorta often presents with hypertension in adults. Discrepancy in the amplitude and timing of the brachial and femoral or popliteal pulse generally indicates significant coarctation. Surgical treatment remains the gold standard, although percutaneous balloon dilatation and stenting are growing in popularity. Hypertension may persist despite surgical correction and will require treatment. All patients with coarctation of the aorta, even following surgical correction, should continue follow-up as aneurysm formation and recurrence of coarctation may occur.

Further Reading

Aboulhosn J, Child JS. Left ventricular outflow obstruction: subaortic stenosis, bicuspid aortic valve, supravalvular aortic stenosis and coarctation of the aorta. *Circulation* 2006; **114**: 2412–22.

Jenkins NP, Ward C. Coarctation of the aorta: natural history and outcome after surgical treatment. *QJM* 1999; **92**: 365–71.

35 Contraception in congenital heart disease

Case History

A 33-year-old woman with a history of 'hole in the heart' is planning to start a family and attended her general practitioner for advice regarding pregnancy. She had a successful procedure to close the hole about 8 years ago. She has been completely asymptomatic and she has no other past medical history of note. On examination, her blood pressure and heart sounds were normal. There was no evidence of cyanosis or heart failure. The patient is keen to start a family soon, but wants to know what the potential implications are for her.

How do you classify the maternal risk of pregnancy?

What contraceptive advice would you offer a patient with heart disease?

Background

The above scenario is increasingly common. About 250 000 adults have congenital heart disease within the UK and this number is increasing as improvements in surgical techniques result in better survival. About half of these patients are women and many are of reproductive age. Cardiac death is a major cause of maternal deaths in the UK, and the risk of death associated with pregnancy is related to the nature of the heart disease. Therefore, all patients with heart disease should be offered adequate pre-conception counselling to avoid unplanned pregnancy (which exposes the mother to the risk of pregnancy) and to inform the mother of the risks associated with the pregnancy. Indeed, all women with heart disease should be offered advice early (e.g. in adolescence) to allow some women to come to terms with their limited child-bearing potential. Patients at high risk of death associated with pregnancy should be offered advice on contraception.

The use of contraceptive methods has been classified by the World Health Organization (WHO) and this classification has been adapted to include the maternal risk of pregnancy and the risk of contraceptive methods for different cardiac conditions (Table 35.1). A number of conditions are not associated with increased maternal risks in the absence of risk factors (e.g. cyanosis, symptoms > NYHA [New York Heart Association] class II, left ventricular ejection fraction <40% and previous cardiovascular complications such as arrhythmias, stroke or thromboembolism) and pregnancy may be advised. On the other extreme, maternal mortality may be as high as 50% in some condi-

Table 35.1 WHO classification

WHO class	Risk of contraceptive method	Maternal risk
1 (always useable)	No higher than general population	No higher than general population
2 (broadly useable)	Small increase in risk, outweighed by advantages	Significant increase in risk. Expert cardiac and obstetric pre-pregnancy, antenatal and postnatal care recommended
3 (use with caution)	Risks outweigh advantages. Use alternatives unless: • Patient accepts risks and rejects alternatives • Risk of pregnancy very high and alternatives not adequately effective	Significant increase in risk. Expert cardiac and obstetric pre-pregnancy required
4 (contraindicated)	Contraindicated	Pregnancy contraindicated or termination should be discussed. Otherwise, expert care required as above

tions and the patient should be advised against pregnancy or termination should be discussed. In most cases, estimation of maternal risk in patients with heart disease will need to be individualized (Table 35.2).

In this case, the patient is asymptomatic. Review of her previous records revealed a history of secundum atrial septal defect, which was successfully closed percutaneously. There was no evidence of pulmonary hypertension. Therefore, this patient's risk from pregnancy is no greater than the general population.

What contraceptive advice would you offer a patient with heart disease?

The use of different contraceptive methods in patients with heart disease should be considered in the context of the risk of the method to the patient and the failure rate of the

Table 35.2 Pregnancy risk

WHO 1	WHO 2	WHO 3	WHO 4
Uncomplicated VSD, PDA	Unoperated ASD	Mechanical heart valve	Pulmonary hypertension
Mild valvular disease	Repaired tetralogy of Fallot	Systemic right ventricle (e.g. congenitally corrected transposition)	Severe LV dysfunction with NYHA III or IV
Repaired secundum ASD, VSD, PDA	Most arrhythmias	Fontan circulation	Severe left heart obstruction (e.g. severe aortic stenosis)
Isolated atrial or ventricular ectopics	Mild LV impairment* Hypertrophic cardiomyopathy* Non-WHO 4 valve disease* Marfan syndrome without aortic dilatation*	Cyanotic heart disease Other complex congenital heart disease	Marfan syndrome with aortic dilatation (>40 mm)

*Some of these patients may be WHO 3 dependent.
ASD, atrial septal defect; LV, left ventricular; PDA, patent ductus arteriosus; VSD, ventricular septal defect.

method (Figure 35.1). Failure rate is a particularly important consideration for patients who would be at high risk of morbidity and mortality if exposed to pregnancy.

The safest contraceptive method, although not necessarily the most effective, is the barrier method (e.g. a condom). It also has the advantage of preventing sexually transmitted disease. It has a significant failure rate and is generally not appropriate for patients who would be at high risk with pregnancy.

Combined (oestrogen and progestogen) oral contraceptives are generally effective but carry an increased risk of thromboembolism. They are therefore contraindicated (WHO 4) in patients with thrombogenic mechanical heart valve (e.g. single leaflet tilting disc) and cyanotic heart disease. The latter suggests the presence of right-to-left shunting, which may allow potentially catastrophic paradoxical embolism (embolism from the venous to the arterial circulation). Patients with other types of mechanical heart valves, previous history of thromboembolism, atrial fibrillation and potential right-to-left shunting (without cyanosis) should be offered alternative contraceptive methods (i.e. WHO 3). Of note, combined oral contraceptives interact with warfarin and close monitoring of anticoagulation is required.

In contrast, the risk of thromboembolism does not appear to be significantly elevated by progestogen-only preparations. Oral progestogen preparations (e.g. Cerazette and Levonelle) are therefore suitable for most patients with heart disease (WHO 1) and offer an effective alternative to combined oral contraceptives. Some oral progestogen preparations may be associated with menstrual irregularities although prolonged use may be associated with amenorrhoea (potentially advantageous in patients with cyanosis or anticoagulation therapy).

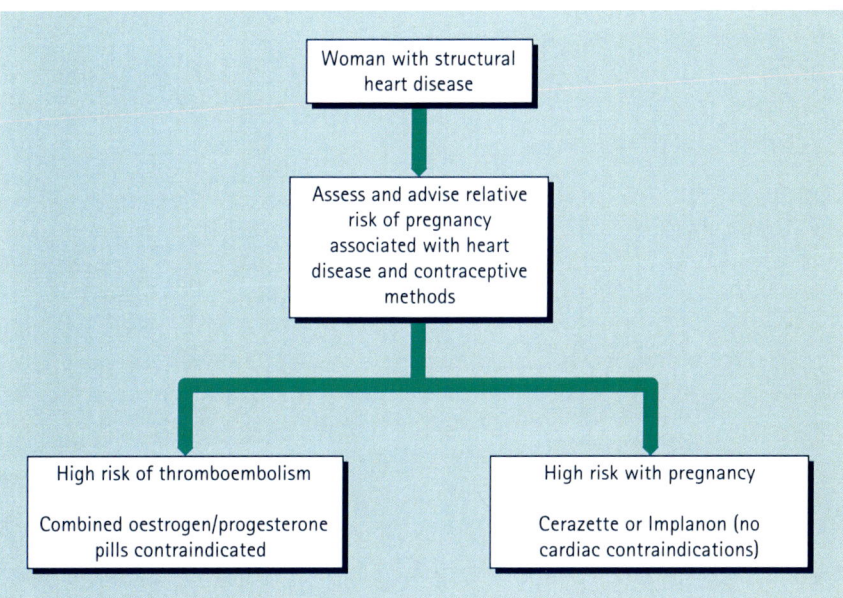

Figure 35.1 Contraception in heart disease.

Other progestogen preparations include Depo Provera, Mirena intrauterine device and Implanon. Depo Provera is an intramuscular injection (every 12 weeks), which is highly effective. However, interruption in treatment may result in rapid return of fertility. The intramuscular injections may also be associated with haematoma in patients on anticoagulation treatment. The Mirena intrauterine device is impregnated with levenorgestrel and is highly effective. It requires replacement every 5 years. Mirena devices usually result in oligo- or amenorrhoea, which may be advantageous. However, implantation of the device may precipitate a vasovagal response in some women, with a catastrophic drop in filling pressures and may be fatal in patients with a Fontan circulation (dependent on high systemic venous pressure to maintain circulation) and pulmonary hypertension. Hence, a Mirena intrauterine device is considered WHO 3 (i.e. use with caution and alternative method if possible) in these patients. The risk of vasovagal response may be reduced by spinal and epidural block. There is also a risk of endocarditis with implantation of the device.

Implanon is a subdermal implant, which is highly effective for up to 3 years. It offers an alternative to the Mirena intrauterine device in patients with Fontan circulation and pulmonary hypertension. However, it may result in troublesome irregular menstrual bleeding. It is generally safe in most patients (WHO 1).

More invasive methods include female sterilization, which although intuitively attractive is actually not as effective as Implanon or the Mirena intrauterine device. Laparoscopic sterilization carries significant risk to some patients, particularly patients with Fontan circulation or pulmonary hypertension, as abdominal insufflation during laparoscopy can significantly reduce venous return and compromise cardiac output. There is also a risk of air embolism and paradoxical embolism in patients with uncorrected shunts. In addition, there is a risk of late failure. Sterilization should therefore be considered WHO 2 in most patients and WHO 3 in patients with Fontan circulation and pulmonary hypertension. Sterilization of the male partner is rarely appropriate as he may outlive his female partner with heart disease.

Conclusion

Some but not all patients with heart disease have an increased risk of morbidity and mortality from pregnancy. Careful evaluation of risk is crucial, as women at low risk should not be denied the opportunity to start a family, while pregnancy may be undesirable in patients at high risk. Contraceptive advice is closely allied to and should be part of this risk assessment. In patients in whom pregnancy risk is high, methods that are more effective are desirable. Patients at moderate to high risk with pregnancy should be referred to a specialist cardiologist and obstetrician for pre-pregnancy, antenatal and postnatal care.

Further Reading

Kovasc AH, Harrison JL, Colman M, *et al*. Pregnancy and contraception in congenital heart disease: what women are not told. *J Am Coll Cardiol* 2008; **52**: 577–8.

Thorne S, MacGregor A, Nelson-Piercy C. Risks of contraception and pregnancy in heart disease. *Heart* 2006; **92**: 1520–5.

Uebing A, Steer PJ, Yentis SM, Gatzoulis MA. Pregnancy and congenital heart disease. *BMJ* 2006; **332**: 401–6.

SECTION EIGHT   08

Pregnancy and Heart Disease

36	Valve disease and pregnancy
37	Prosthetic valve and anticoagulation
38	Hypertension in pregnancy

PROBLEM

36 Valve disease and pregnancy

Case History

A 30-year-old woman from Pakistan presented to the medical services 25 weeks into her first pregnancy with increasing breathlessness on minimal effort. On further inquiry, she complained of worsening orthopnoea and paroxysmal nocturnal dyspnoea. She denied any chest pain. Before her pregnancy, she had good exercise tolerance with only minor breathlessness on exertion. Her past medical history is not clear. On examination, her respiratory rate was 36 breaths/minute at rest, with a resting heart rate of 140 beats/minute with oxygen saturations of 94% on air. Her blood pressure was 110/80 mmHg. The heart sounds were difficult to assess due to the tachycardia, but there was a suggestion of a diastolic murmur. There were crackles in both lung bases. Her electrocardiogram confirmed sinus tachycardia with no significant ST segment changes.

How would you assess this patient?

How do the physiological changes in pregnancy affect a patient with mitral stenosis?

What are the risks of mitral stenosis in pregnancy?

How would you manage mitral stenosis in pregnancy?

Background

Clinically, this patient is in heart failure. Potential causes include a pre-existing cardiomyopathy, valvular dysfunction or congenital heart disease exacerbated by the haemodynamic changes in pregnancy, a new-onset cardiomyopathy (e.g. peripartum cardiomyopathy or myocarditis) and a consequence of acute myocardial infarction. In this case, the patient's previous medical history is not clear but there was a suggestion of a diastolic murmur. This should raise the suspicion of valvular heart disease. Peripartum cardiomyopathy typically occurs in the latter stages of a pregnancy but should be excluded. The clinical presentation is not typical of acute myocardial infarction.

Transthoracic echocardiography is a useful non-invasive investigation. In this case, the left ventricular dimensions and systolic function were normal, but the left atrium was dilated. There was thickening of the mitral valve with reduced valve excursion. There was also thickening of the subvalvular apparatus. The mitral valve area was moderately stenosed with an estimated area of 1.1 cm^2. There was only mild mitral regurgitation and mild thickening of the aortic valve. The changes were suggestive of rheumatic mitral stenosis. Mitral stenosis is the most common valve disease in pregnancy and is usually a result of rheumatic heart disease. Although the incidence of rheumatic heart disease has declined significantly in developed countries, it remains prevalent in developing countries.

How do the physiological changes in pregnancy affect a patient with mitral stenosis?

Pregnancy induces a number of physiological changes. Plasma volume is increased by up to 50% by 32 weeks of gestation, with activation of the renin–angiotensin system. The increase in plasma volume exceeds the increase in red cell mass, resulting in dilutional anaemia. Cardiac output in the healthy mother increases in proportion with increases in plasma volume but tends to peak at about 16 weeks. Despite the increase in cardiac output, blood pressure typically drops due to significant vasodilatation. Other changes include an increase in insulin resistance, which may precipitate gestational diabetes and increase in thrombotic tendency (increase in procoagulants and reduced fibrinolytic activity).

In a patient with fixed obstruction on the left side of the heart, the increase in plasma volume may not be matched by a similar increase in cardiac output. In a patient with mitral stenosis, the left atrial pressure increases due to the fixed stenosis of the mitral valve, and this in turn increases pulmonary venous pressure and pulmonary congestion. The increase in left atrial pressure may be exacerbated by tachycardia as the time interval for diastolic transmitral flow is shortened at faster heart rates. Often, the increase in left atrial pressure may precipitate atrial fibrillation, which may significantly increase the risk of thromboembolism (particularly with the hypercoagulable state in pregnancy).

What are the risks of mitral stenosis in pregnancy?

Mitral stenosis carries a risk to both the mother and the foetus. The risks are linked to the severity of the stenosis and the functional status prior to the pregnancy. A number of studies have reported on the outcome of pregnancies in mothers with mitral stenosis. In general, maternal outcome in mild mitral stenosis is comparable with normal pregnancies. In one study, the incidence of maternal complications (pulmonary oedema and atrial arrhythmias) was reported to be as high as 67% in patients with severe mitral stenosis and 38% with moderate mitral stenosis. Overall, maternal deaths are uncommon in patients with mitral stenosis (few reports of deaths in patients with severe mitral stenosis and New York Heart Association class [NYHA] III/IV). Adverse foetal outcomes include premature delivery, intrauterine growth retardation and low birth weight. In one study, premature delivery (28% in moderate stenosis versus 6% in controls, 44% in severe stenosis versus 11% in controls) and intrauterine growth retardation (27% in moderate stenosis, 33% in severe stenosis versus 0% in controls) are significantly higher in patients with moderate or severe mitral stenosis.

How would you manage mitral stenosis in pregnancy?

All women with heart disease should be offered counselling prior to conception. In some patients with symptomatic severe mitral stenosis, percutaneous balloon mitral valvuloplasty may be contemplated before conception. Mitral valve replacement prior to conception may not be appropriate as this may expose the mother and the foetus to risks associated with a prosthetic valve in pregnancy. Pregnancy with significant valve disease should be managed by specialist cardiologists and obstetricians.

In this case, the patient is already pregnant and presenting with progressive heart failure. Treatment in these cases should be aimed at controlling heart rate and reducing left atrial pressure. Control of heart rate may be achieved by bed rest, restricting physical activity and rate-lowering drugs. β-blockers, particularly with $β_1$ selectivity (to avoid antagonism of $β_2$-mediated uterine relaxation), such as metoprolol, are preferred. There are some reports of intrauterine growth retardation with atenolol. Higher doses may be required due to the increased sympathetic activity in pregnancy. In patients intolerant of β-blockers, verapamil may be used instead. There are some reports of birth defects with diltiazem, particularly if used in the first trimester. Digoxin may be added in patients with atrial fibrillation. Anticoagulation should also be considered in patients with atrial fibrillation. Salt restriction and oral diuretic treatment may reduce left atrial pressure. Diuretic treatment should be carefully titrated to avoid over-diuresis, which may compromise uteroplacental perfusion.

Medical treatment alone may be successful in most cases. However, in patients with severe mitral stenosis and persistent NYHA class III/IV symptoms despite medical therapy, percutaneous balloon mitral valvuloplasty may be considered. Small studies suggest that this procedure may be safe although clinical experience remains limited in pregnancy. Mitral valve surgery should only be considered as the last resort as this is associated with significant maternal mortality and even higher rates of foetal loss.

A number of studies have also reported on the mode of delivery. In general, vaginal delivery with a shortened second stage (e.g. with forceps) can be tolerated by most women with mitral stenosis. Caesarean section may be considered for obstetric indications. Epidural anaesthesia may minimize fluctuations in cardiac output and is generally recommended. Hypotension associated with epidural anaesthesia may be managed with vasoconstrictors (without positive chronotropic effect) and crystalloid. All patients should be closely monitored throughout and after delivery, as increased venous return early in the puerperium may precipitate pulmonary oedema. In this case, the patient was treated with β-blockers and oral diuretics. She had an uncomplicated vaginal delivery.

Recent Developments

The traditional view that regional anaesthesia (e.g. epidural) is contraindicated in patients with heart disease is outdated. In general, adequate (regional) analgesia coupled with (assisted) vaginal delivery is associated with more favourable haemodynamics than Caesarean section in women with valvular heart disease. Effective management of heart disease in pregnancy requires a specialist multidisciplinary team approach.

Conclusion

Mitral stenosis is the most common valvular disease in pregnancy. It is usually rheumatic in aetiology. Maternal and foetal complications are related to the severity of the stenosis. Medical treatment with bed rest, rate control and diuretic therapy is usually successful. Percutaneous balloon mitral valvuloplasty may occasionally be required in patients with refractory symptoms despite medical treatment.

Further Reading

Elkayam U, Bitar F. Valvular heart disease and pregnancy: native valves. *J Am Coll Cardiol* 2005; **46**: 223–30.

Thorne SA. Pregnancy in heart disease. *Heart* 2004; **90**: 450–6.

PROBLEM

37 Prosthetic valve and anticoagulation

Case History

A 30-year-old woman with a mechanical aortic valve has just had a positive pregnancy test. She is normally on warfarin. She is keen to continue with the pregnancy, but is concerned about her heart valve and the effects of warfarin on her baby. She is asymptomatic. On examination, she had a clear prosthetic first heart sound with a soft systolic flow murmur. There was no evidence of heart failure.

How would you assess this patient?

How would you manage anticoagulation for a mechanical valve in pregnancy?

Are bioprosthetic valves preferable to mechanical valves in women of child-bearing age?

Background

In general, women with heart disease should receive counselling prior to conception to inform them of the risks of pregnancy. In this case, the patient should be made aware of the need for anticoagulation treatment during pregnancy and associated risks. An echocardiogram to assess the valve and other potential abnormalities may provide a useful baseline assessment. These patients should be referred to specialist cardiologists and obstetricians for antenatal and postnatal care.

How would you manage anticoagulation for a mechanical valve in pregnancy?

Anticoagulation treatment in a pregnant woman is a balance of risks: risk of inadequate anticoagulation (e.g. valve thrombosis), risk of bleeding in the mother and risk to the foetus (teratogenicity and foetal loss). In the case of a prosthetic valve, the risk without anticoagulation is dependent on the type and location of the prosthetic valve. Older (e.g. Bjork–Shiley and Starr–Edwards) prosthetic valves in the mitral position carry a high risk of thrombosis without anticoagulation, while the risk of thrombosis is lower with newer bileaflet valves, particularly in the aortic position. The risk of valve thrombosis may be accentuated in pregnancy due to the hypercoagulable state. Warfarin is more effective than heparin in reducing the risk of valve thrombosis. There are suggestions that unfractionated heparins may be more effective than low molecular weight heparins, but the latter are used in the management of prosthetic valves in pregnancy, with anti-factor Xa activity monitoring (to ensure efficacy), by some centres in the UK.

The risk of bleeding can be minimized with close monitoring of anticoagulation therapy (warfarin or heparin). Indeed, the safest option for the mother is to remain on warfarin throughout the pregnancy, stopped for 2 weeks before a planned elective Caesarean section with heparin cover. As warfarin crosses the placenta, the baby may be anticoagulated and exposed to an increased risk of bleeding during delivery even when delivery is by Caesarean section (heparin does not cross the placenta).

However, warfarin is associated with 'warfarin embryopathy' (nasal hypoplasia and stippled epiphyses). The incidence of 'warfarin embryopathy' has been variably reported, but appears to be about 7% (and may be even higher) of live births if warfarin is used throughout pregnancy or restricted to the second and third trimesters. The incidence of 'warfarin embryopathy' may be reduced if heparin is used in the first 3 months (particularly between 6 and 12 weeks of pregnancy). Hence, based on these considerations, one recommended approach may be to replace warfarin with heparin in the first 6–12 weeks and the last 2 weeks of pregnancy to reduce the risk of embryopathy, protect the mother against thrombotic complications and minimize the risk of bleeding. Warfarin should be recommenced after delivery as the risk of thrombosis remains in the post-partum period. The choice of heparin is controversial, with unfractionated heparin recommended in the USA but low molecular weight heparin (with anti-factor Xa monitoring) favoured in the UK.

In this case, the patient was treated with low molecular weight heparin with anti-factor Xa monitoring during the first 3 months, followed by her regular warfarin therapy, followed by low molecular weight heparin in the last 2 weeks. Warfarin was restarted thereafter. Of note, warfarin is safe in breastfeeding.

Are bioprosthetic valves preferable to mechanical valves in women of child-bearing age?

Bioprosthetic valves can be classified as heterografts, homografts and autografts. Example of a heterograft is the Carpentier–Edwards porcine bioprosthesis. Homografts may offer superior haemodynamics compared with porcine valves and may have lower rates of infection. The Ross procedure, which replaces the diseased aortic valve with the patient's own pulmonary valve, is an example of autograft. Some reports suggest excellent durability with the Ross procedure. However, the Ross procedure is technically more demanding and may be associated with higher perioperative mortality. Bioprosthetic valves do not require long-term anticoagulation treatment.

Bioprosthetic valves, which obviate the need for anticoagulation treatment, may seem to be the obvious choice for young women of child-bearing age. However, structural valve deterioration is a major limitation with these bioprosthetic heart valves, particularly in younger patients and in the mitral position. Significant valve deterioration may occur within 2–3 years and may be as high as 50% in 10 years in young patients, which contrasts with the excellent durability of the current bileaflet mechanical valves. Mortality from reoperation may be as high as 5%. There is no clear evidence that homografts or autografts are superior to porcine bioprosthetic valves in terms of structural valve deterioration or mortality from reoperation. Several reports also suggest that the haemodynamic burden associated with pregnancy may accelerate structural valve deterioration, although this has not been a consistent finding. Data for homografts and autografts in pregnancy are very limited. Nonetheless, regular monitoring of valve function, clinically and by echocardiography, is recommended.

Hence, there are significant limitations to both mechanical and bioprosthetic valves and the choice of valve prosthesis should be made after close discussion between the surgeon, the cardiologist and, most importantly, the patient.

Recent Developments

The use of low molecular weight heparin in pregnant women with prosthetic heart valves has been controversial, not least due to the warning issued by the manufacturer. Recent guidelines have not rejected the use of low molecular weight heparins for this indication but emphasize the importance of monitoring levels of factor Xa.

Conclusion

Management of a pregnant woman with mechanical heart valve is difficult and requires a balancing of risks to both the mother and the baby. The woman should be informed of these risks before conception, and the antenatal and postnatal care should be managed by specialist cardiologists and obstetricians. The choice of prosthetic valve in young patients is similarly complex and bioprosthetic valves are not necessarily the 'safer' option for women contemplating pregnancy.

Further Reading

Hung L, Rahimtoola SH. Prosthetic heart valves and pregnancy. *Circulation* 2003; **107**: 1240–6.

Thorne SA. Pregnancy in heart disease. *Heart* 2004; **90**: 450–6.

PROBLEM

38 Hypertension in pregnancy

Case History

A 34-year-old Afro-Caribbean woman attended a routine antenatal assessment at 12 weeks gestation and was found to have a blood pressure of 150/92 mmHg. She has no previous diagnosis of hypertension or any other medical illness. She is an ex-smoker and does not take any regular medications. On examination, she was overweight and her cardiovascular examination was normal. Urine dipstick did not reveal any proteinuria. The midwife is concerned about the blood pressure and asks for your advice.

How would you classify hypertension in pregnancy?

How would you manage hypertension in pregnancy?

How would you manage this patient following the pregnancy?

Background

Normal or acceptable blood pressure is generally regarded as <140/90 mmHg. Mild-to-moderate hypertension is defined as <160/110 mmHg and severe hypertension as >160/110 mmHg. Hypertension in pregnancy may fall into one of four groups complicating chronic hypertension.

1. Chronic or pre-existing hypertension.
2. Gestational hypertension.
3. Pre-eclampsia/eclampsia.
4. Pre-eclampsia.

The diagnosis of chronic or pre-existing hypertension requires either recognition of hypertension prior to gestation or failure of hypertension to resolve following pregnancy (generally if blood pressure of >140/90 mmHg persists 3 months postpartum). Similarly, gestational hypertension may be diagnosed in a woman known not to have pre-existing hypertension or if hypertension resolves postpartum (i.e. diagnosed retrospectively). Gestational hypertension complicates about 6% of pregnancies and tends to occur in the latter half of the pregnancy. Patients with gestational hypertension are at increased risk of pre-eclampsia, particularly if there is a previous history of miscarriages or hypertension during pregnancy. The patient in this case is likely to have chronic or pre-existing hypertension.

Pre-eclampsia/eclampsia is characterized by hypertension (either new-onset or complicating pre-existing hypertension) after 20 weeks of gestation (usually closer to term) and associated proteinuria. This syndrome occurs in up to 8% of pregnancies and is believed to be a result of abnormal vasculature in the placenta, impaired placental perfusion and release of various growth/angiogenic factors into the systemic circulation. The syndrome may be complicated by neurological (occipital headaches and seizures) and hepatic (deranged liver function tests and reduced platelet count) involvement. Uncontrolled hypertension may also result in target organ damage and cerebral haemorrhage. Of note, women with gestational hypertension are at increased risk of pre-eclampsia, which may occur in the first week postpartum. Hence, blood pressure monitoring is required in the postpartum period.

Other maternal risk factors for pre-eclampsia include first pregnancy, age younger than 18 years or older than 35 years, chronic hypertension, personal or family history of pre-eclampsia, pre-gestational diabetes, obesity and renal dysfunction. Foetal risk factors include multiple gestations, molar pregnancies, hydrops and triploidy. A Cochrane review suggests that aspirin may reduce the risk of developing pre-eclampsia and the associated adverse outcomes.

How would you manage hypertension in pregnancy?

The treatment of hypertension in pregnancy necessarily differs from conventional treatment of blood pressure. First, the classification of hypertension in pregnancy deviates from the conventional classification of blood pressure. Diastolic rather than systolic blood pressure is often emphasized in pregnancy. Second, the blood pressure treatment target differs from conventional hypertension. Third, the primary objective of blood pressure treatment in pregnancy is maternal and foetal safety (i.e. safety over 9 months rather than years).

A number of clinical studies have shown higher risks of placental abruption, accelerated hypertension with target organ damage and cerebral haemorrhage in mothers with hypertension during pregnancy. Adverse foetal outcomes such as growth retardation and prematurity are also more common in women with hypertension. While blood pressure lowering in patients with severe hypertension (>160/110 mmHg) with or without pre-eclampsia, may reduce maternal complications, the value of treating mild-to-moderate hypertension is less well established. Recent meta-analyses suggest that antihypertensive treatment in patients with mild-to-moderate hypertension may reduce the risk of progressing to severe hypertension but there is no difference in pre-eclampsia or foetal outcomes. Blood pressure in some women with pre-existing mild-to-moderate hypertension may even fall during pregnancy due to physiological vasodilatation. The uncertain value of antihypertensive treatment in patients with mild-to-moderate hypertension has led to varying recommendations, with some recommending treatment only in patients with blood pressure of >160/110 mmHg and others suggesting treatment if blood pressure >150/90 mmHg. The patient in this case has mild-to-moderate chronic hypertension with no evidence of target organ damage early in her pregnancy. A decision was made to defer antihypertensive therapy and keep her under close review (Figure 38.1).

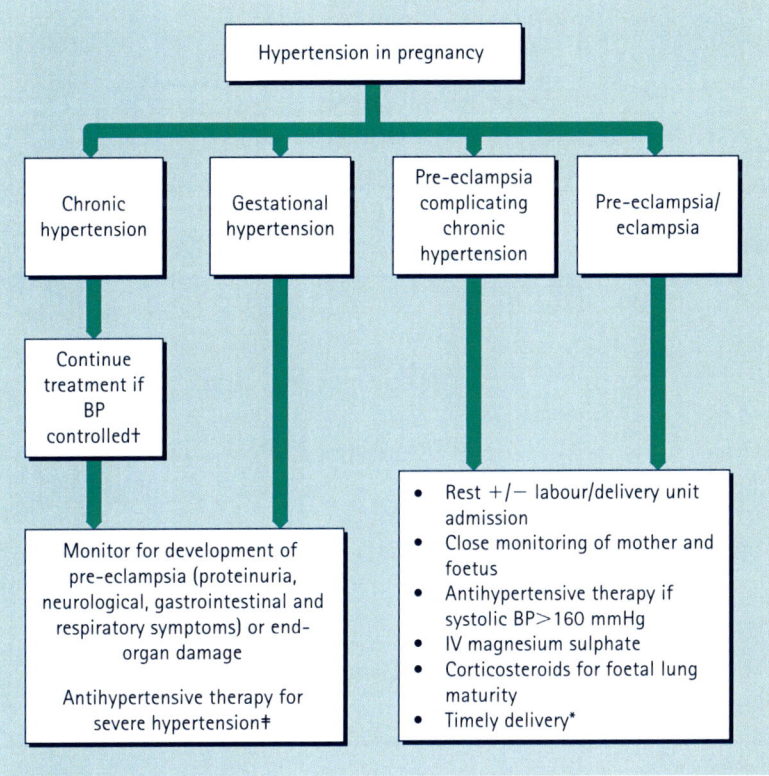

Figure 38.1 Hypertension in pregnancy. BP, blood pressure. [*]Overall management is dependent on maternal and foetal considerations, particularly the severity of pre-eclampsia/eclampsia and gestation; †except for treatments associated with terotogenicity (e.g. angiotensin-converting enzyme inhibitors, angiotensin receptor blockers); ‡oral therapy usually sufficient.

The choice of antihypertensive therapy depends on maternal comorbidities, the presence of complications associated with hypertension and the stage of pregnancy. Pre-eclampsia at term should be delivered with blood pressure monitoring/treatment in the peri- and postpartum period. The choice of antihypertensive agents in pregnancy is limited by potential teratogenicity. Angiotensin-converting enzyme inhibitors and angiotensin receptor blockers are contraindicated due to risk of oligohydramnios and renal dysgenesis. Spironolactone has anti-androgenic effects and should not be used in pregnancy. There are some reports of low birth weight with atenolol but there are no reports of teratogenicity. Intravenous β-blocker treatment may result in clinically significant foetal bradycardia. β-blockers may be contraindicated in mothers with asthma. Antihypertensive agents used in pregnancy are listed in Table 38.1. In contrast to the abundance of data to guide therapy in conventional hypertension, data on the use of antihypertensive treatment are generally limited to case series, observation data or small studies.

Oral treatment is sufficient and indeed preferred in the majority of cases (even in severe hypertension), unless there is associated target organ damage (e.g. encephalopathy

Table 38.1 Antihypertensive agents used in pregnancy	
Methyldopa	Favoured treatment in gestational/chronic hypertension. Good clinical experience, documented safety after first trimester
Labetolol	Oral therapy as effective as methyldopa. Probably parenteral agent of choice as lower incidence of significant hypotension. Can cause foetal bradycardia, especially if administered parenterally. Possible foetal growth restriction. Contraindicated in patients with asthma
Other β-blockers	Risk of growth retardation if used in the first/second trimester (particularly atenolol)
Nifedipine	Favoured calcium channel blocker based on clinical experience. May inhibit labour. Use slow-release preparation only
Hydralazine	Good clinical experience. Parenteral use in severe hypertension may be associated with significant hypotension and foetal distress (labetolol preferred). Neonatal thrombocytopaenia reported. Can cause headaches, nausea and vomiting (i.e. mimics eclampsia)
Thiazide diuretics	Potential adverse metabolic (glucose intolerance). Alter serum uric acid (hence unreliable in pre-eclampsia)
Sodium nitroprusside	Parenteral agent if other therapy unsuccessful. Cyanate toxicity if >24–48 hours of use (especially in renal/hepatic dysfunction)

and cerebral haemorrhage) or eclampsia, when parenteral treatment is indicated. Intravenous labetolol is generally preferred over hydralazine if parenteral treatment is required, as labetolol is associated with a lower risk of significant hypotension. Women with pre-eclampsia, in particular, are often volume depleted and may be more susceptible to the hypotensive effects of vasodilators. Treatment should be initiated cautiously to avoid a precipitous drop in blood pressure, which may compromise uteroplacental blood flow. Sodium nitroprusside, which is widely used in hypertensive emergencies tends to be reserved for refractory hypertension. Foetal monitoring is essential during treatment. The treatment of eclampsia is beyond the scope of this chapter.

There are no specific studies to guide blood pressure treatment targets in pregnancy. In general, in patients with severe hypertension requiring parenteral treatment, blood pressure should be lowered gradually (e.g. 25% reduction in mean blood pressure in the first hour). Immediate normalization of blood pressure may be detrimental to the mother and foetus (placental and foetal hypoperfusion). Similarly, a safe or ideal blood pressure target (if it exists) in pregnancy is unknown. In general, blood pressure lowering with oral treatment to the range of 140–150/90–100 mmHg in patients with pre-eclampsia or severe uncomplicated hypertension may be reasonable. As some patients with mild-to-moderate hypertension may 'normalize' their blood pressure during pregnancy, antihypertensive treatment may not always be necessary, particularly as it has not been shown to improve maternal or foetal outcomes in these patients.

How would you manage this patient following the pregnancy?

Patients with hypertension during pregnancy should be monitored in the postpartum period as there remains a risk of pre-eclampsia in some patients with gestational hypertension. Patients with persistent hypertension at least 3 months postpartum are likely to have chronic hypertension and should be managed in accordance with current recommendations for hypertension. Hypertension during pregnancy should be clearly documented as these patients have an increased risk of pre-eclampsia in future pregnancies.

Unlike treatment during pregnancy, a large number of antihypertensive agents are safe in breastfeeding (Table 38.2). Notably, angiotensin-converting enzyme inhibitors, which are contraindicated in pregnancy, may be compatible with breastfeeding (enalapril and captopril). In contrast, some drugs used in pregnancy (e.g. atenolol) may be concentrated in breast milk and thus incompatible with breastfeeding.

Table 38.2 Some antihypertensive agents compatible with breastfeeding

- Captopril
- Enalapril
- Labetolol
- Methyldopa
- Hydralazine
- Hydrochlorothiazide
- Diltiazem
- Verapamil
- Nifedipine
- Spironolactone

Recent Developments

Blood pressure control during pregnancy has been the subject of a small pilot study that included 132 women with non-proteinuric pre-existing or gestational hypertension, randomized to either tight (target diastolic blood pressure 85 mmHg) or less tight (target diastolic blood pressure 100 mmHg). This study suggests that serious maternal and perinatal complications may not be higher in patients with less tight blood pressure control. Future studies will evaluate potential blood pressure treatment targets in pregnancy.

Conclusion

Hypertension complicates about 10% of pregnancies and can be divided into chronic hypertension, gestational hypertension and pre-eclampsia/eclampsia with or without pre-existing hypertension. In some cases, diagnosis can only be made retrospectively. Oral treatment is sufficient in the majority of patients. Parenteral treatment should be reserved for patients with hypertensive emergencies or eclampsia. Specific blood pressure targets have not been established but gradual blood pressure lowering to 140–150/90–100 mmHg in pre-eclampsia is generally recommended.

Further Reading

Podymow T, August P. Update on the use of antihypertensive drugs in pregnancy. *Hypertension* 2008; **51**: 960–9.

Report of the National High Blood Pressure Education Program Working Group on High Blood Pressure in Pregnancy. *Am J Obstet Gynecol* 2000; **183**: S1–22.

SECTION NINE 09

Cardiac Disease and Operative Risk

39   Perioperative risk stratification and β-blocker

PROBLEM

39 Perioperative risk stratification and β-blocker

Case History

A vascular surgeon reviewed a 72-year-old man with a history of abdominal aortic aneurysm and recommended surgical repair of the aneurysm in view of the risk of aneurysm rupture. The surgeon, however, was concerned about the man's risk of perioperative cardiovascular complications and referred him for a pre-operative assessment. The man is an ex-smoker and has a previous history of myocardial infarction 3 years ago, treated successfully by percutaneous coronary intervention, and he has been free of angina since. His blood pressure appeared to be adequately controlled by a combination of a β-blocker and an angiotensin-converting enzyme inhibitor. He had impaired glucose tolerance but normal renal function. He denied any significant breathlessness and his exercise capacity was limited by osteoarthritis.

How is the risk of perioperative myocardial infarction assessed?

Is there a role for β-blocker treatment to reduce the risk of perioperative myocardial infarction?

Is there a role for coronary angiography and percutaneous coronary intervention prior to surgery?

Background

Perioperative myocardial infarction is a major cause of morbidity and mortality among patients undergoing non-cardiac surgery. In particular, patients undergoing vascular surgery are at high risk due to the high prevalence of significant coronary artery disease, which may be occult or manifest. Pre-operative management of patients undergoing non-cardiac surgery has two main objectives.

1. To assess the risk of perioperative cardiovascular complications (particularly perioperative myocardial infarction and stroke).
2. To optimize/introduce medical treatment/intervention to reduce the risk of perioperative cardiovascular complications.

However, these two objectives of pre-operative management are often difficult to achieve, particularly as robust evidence in support of the latter are lacking.

The initial assessment should be based on clinical history and electrocardiogram (ECG) evaluation, with the aim of identifying the six key clinical variables of the Revised Cardiac Risk Index (RCRI) (Table 39.1). The RCRI has been validated in a number of studies and found to be superior to other risk stratification tools for perioperative assessment of cardiovascular risk.

Exercise and pharmacological stress testing have excellent negative predictive values (i.e. useful for reducing risk estimate when negative or normal) but poor positive predictive values (i.e. may not identify patients at highest risk when positive). Compared with exercise testing, pharmacological stress tests have superior discriminative power and can be used in patients with functional limitations (e.g. patients with claudication) or baseline ECG abnormalities. Where available, dobutamine stress echocardiography may be preferable because of higher specificity and the additional information from echocardiography (left ventricular function and valvular heart disease), which may affect risk estimation.

Is there a role for β-blocker treatment to reduce the risk of perioperative myocardial infarction?

The benefit of perioperative β-blockers has been the subject of a number of studies, with conflicting conclusions. Data from an observational study of almost 700 000 patients suggested that β-blockers given within 2 days of any non-cardiac surgery provided

Table 39.1 The Revised Cardiac Risk Index

High-risk surgical procedure
    Thoracic, abdominal or pelvic vascular (e.g. aorta, renal, mesenteric) surgery

Ischaemic heart disease
    History of myocardial infarction, angina, use of sublingual GTN, positive exercise test, Q waves on ECG, previous percutaneous coronary intervention or coronary artery bypass graft surgery

Heart failure
    From clinical history, examination or chest X-ray

Cerebrovascular disease
    History of stroke or transient ischaemic attack

Diabetes mellitus on insulin therapy

Chronic renal failure
    Creatinine >177 μmol/l

Rates of major cardiac complications (myocardial infarction, pulmonary oedema and cardiac arrest) for 0, 1, 2 or ≥3 estimated to be 0.4%, 0.9%, 7% and 11%. GTN, glyceryl trinitrate.

protective benefit only in patients at higher risk (RCRI>2). In patients at low risk (RCRI of 0 or 1), the use of β-blockers was associated with an increased risk of complications. The recently published Perioperative Ischaemia Evaluation (POISE) trial, which included over 8000 patients with at least one cardiac risk factor, randomized to either extended-release metoprolol or placebo, suggested that extended-release metoprolol might reduce rates of myocardial infarction but at the expense of increased rates of hypotensive and bradycardic episodes, deaths and disabling strokes. Patients already receiving a β-blocker were excluded from this trial. Of note, this trial used a relatively high dose of extended-release metoprolol (100 mg) initiated 2–4 hours before surgery. It is possible that lower doses titrated gradually over days may reduce the rates of hypotension and related complications. Nevertheless, routine perioperative use of β-blockers is not recommended.

Current guidelines (yet to incorporate the findings from the POISE trial) recommend that β-blockers should be continued in patients already taking them, but initiated only for patients identified as at high risk (defined by clinical risk factors or ischaemia on preoperative tests) who are undergoing intermediate or high-risk procedures. In this case, as the patient was already on atenolol, he was advised to continue with the treatment.

Is there a role for coronary angiography and percutaneous coronary intervention prior to surgery?

Patients with high clinical risk (RCRI ≥3), including a background of coronary disease, particularly those with continuing symptoms of angina and/or high-risk features on non-invasive testing, should be considered for coronary angiography. However, there are no randomized trials to support a strategy of 'prophylactic' coronary revascularization to reduce perioperative risk of cardiovascular complications in the absence of conventional indications. The study by McFalls *et al.* (2004) randomized patients with stable angina to either revascularization (either percutaneous coronary intervention or coronary artery bypass graft surgery) or medical treatment and reported no difference in clinical outcomes. This study excluded patients with left main stem disease, ejection fraction <20% and aortic stenosis.

Current guidelines recommend that patients with high clinical risk (RCRI of 3 or more) should be considered for diagnostic coronary angiography, particularly if non-invasive stress testing demonstrates evidence of ischaemia (Figure 39.1). At present, there is no compelling evidence to support 'prophylactic' revascularization, unless there is a conventional established indication for revascularization (e.g. acute coronary syndrome), but revascularization may be appropriate if diagnostic catheterization reveals high-risk conditions (left main disease or multivessel disease with depressed ejection fraction) that excluded these patients from published trials. In this case, this man has a RCRI of 2 (high-risk surgery and history of ischaemic heart disease) with no symptoms of angina. Therefore, he did not undergo further stress testing or coronary angiography. He underwent an uncomplicated surgical repair of his abdominal aneurysm.

The timing of non-cardiac surgery following revascularization represents another area of uncertainty, as routine dual antiplatelet therapy (aspirin and clopidogrel) following percutaneous coronary intervention is associated with an increased risk of bleeding. While surgery soon after balloon angioplasty (within 2 weeks) may be safe, a longer period of dual antiplatelet treatment may be preferable after coronary stenting. As patients with drug-eluting stents are at an increased risk of stent thrombosis for a longer

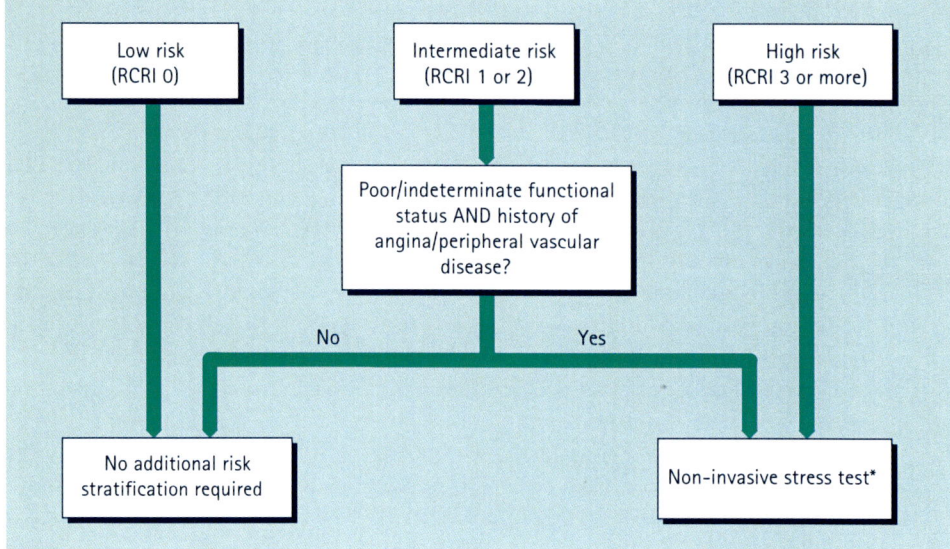

Figure 39.1 Peri-operative risk stratification. β-blocker should be considered only in patients with Revised Cardiac Risk Index (RCRI) of 2 or more. *Cardiac catheterization and revascularization if stress test is positive (refer to text for more detail).

period after stenting compared with bare metal stents, non-cardiac surgery may need to be deferred for a longer period of dual antiplatelet therapy (at least 3–6 months). At present, there are no specific data on how patients with drug-eluting stents should be managed in the perioperative period or how to manage patients who have bare metal stents and require non-cardiac surgery within 6 weeks of stent placement. Discontinuation of clopidogrel is associated with an increased risk of stent thrombosis, particularly in the postoperative setting (increased thrombotic tendency). These cases will need to be evaluated individually (between the surgeon and the cardiologist) and in some cases, perioperative use of short-acting intravenous glycoprotein IIb/IIIa inhibitor may need to be considered.

Recent Developments

Perioperative myocardial infarction may be a consequence of increased oxygen demand in the setting of coronary stenosis and/or *de novo* fissuring of atherosclerotic plaques (even in a non-stenotic segment of the coronary artery) with resultant thrombotic occlusion of the coronary artery. The relative contributions of each of these two mechanisms require further study. Based on data from recent studies, routine β-blocker treatment and 'prophylactic' revascularization cannot be recommended. Non-invasive assessment in high-risk patients may be indicated on the (as yet untested) basis that revascularization may reduce the risk of perioperative myocardial infarction due to coronary stenosis limiting coronary flow in response to increased oxygen demand.

Conclusion

Assessment of perioperative risk of cardiovascular complications should begin with simple clinical evaluation based on the RCRI. A pharmacological stress test (e.g. dobutamine stress echocardiogram) should be considered in patients at high or (symptomatic) intermediate risk, particularly in patients with limited exercise capacity (e.g. due to claudication). The absence of ischaemia on stress testing is reassuring and the patient may proceed with surgery, but coronary angiography should be considered if the stress test is positive with a view to revascularization, particularly in the presence of prognostically significant coronary disease (e.g. left main stem disease). There is no clear evidence to support revascularization in cases of more favourable coronary anatomy (particularly in the absence of angina) and cases will need to be evaluated individually. β-blockers should not be used routinely in patients undergoing surgery.

Further Reading

Auerbach A, Goldman L. Assessing and reducing the cardiac risk of noncardiac surgery. *Circulation* 2006; **113**: 1361–76.

Lee TH, Marcantonio ER, Mangione CM, *et al*. Derivation and prospective validation of a simple index for prediction of cardiac risk of major noncardiac surgery. *Circulation* 1999; **100**: 1043–9.

McFalls EO, Ward HB, Moritz TE, *et al*. Coronary-artery revascularization before elective major vascular surgery. *N Engl J Med* 2004; **351**: 2795–804.

Index

4S (Scandinavian Simvastatin Survival Study) 61

abciximab, in facilitation of PCI 43
accessory pathways 108
ACCORD (Action to Control Cardiovascular Risk in Diabetes) trial 10
ACE (angiotensin-converting enzyme) inhibitors
   ALLHAT 7–8
   avoidance during pregnancy 191
   in dilated cardiomyopathy 145
   in hypertension 72
   indications and contraindications 8
   in mitral regurgitation 89
   in secondary prevention 62
   in stable angina 27
   in STEMI 42
acute coronary syndrome 30, 36
   diagnostic algorithm 31
   risk stratification 31–2
   see also myocardial infarction; non-ST elevation myocardial infarction (NSTEMI); ST elevation myocardial infarction (STEMI)
adenosine
   in stress testing 20
   in termination of supraventricular tachycardias 110
ADVANCE (Action in Diabetes and Vascular Disease: Preterax and Diamicron MR Controlled Evaluation) study 10, 60
AL amyloidosis 150
   see also amyloidosis
alcohol septal ablation 140
aldosterone receptor antagonists
   in secondary prevention 62
   in STEMI 42
aliskiren 10
ALLHAT (Antihypertensive and Lipid-Lowering Treatment to Prevent Heart Attack Trial) 7–8
alpha-blockers
   ALLHAT 7–8
   indications and contraindications 8
aminophylline
   in bradyarrhythmias 127
   in peri-infarct arrhythmias 54–5
amiodarone
   in atrial fibrillation 58, 115, 117
   in peri-infarct arrhythmias 56
   pharmacological cardioversion 116
   in supraventricular tachycardias 111
   in ventricular tachycardias 122, 123
amlodipine 9
   ALLHAT 7–8
   in hypertension 72
   in NSTEMI 35
   in stable angina 26
amyloidosis
   biopsy 149
   echocardiography 147–8
   further investigations 150
   imaging 149–50
   treatment 150
Anderson–Fabry disease 141
angina
   ACE inhibitors 27
   angiography 22
   antiplatelet agents 24
   beta-blockers 25
   calcium channel blockers 26
   causes 18
   clinical presentation 17
   coronary artery bypass grafting 28
   COURAGE trial 28–9
   initial investigations 18–19
   ivabradine 26
   lipid-lowering medication 27
   nitrates 26
   percutaneous transluminal coronary angioplasty 28
   potassium channel agonists 26
   ranolazine 26
   risk factors for 18
   stress testing 20–2
   symptom severity classification 18, 19
   treatment algorithm 25
   treatment following angiography 27
   see also unstable angina
angiography see coronary angiography
angioplasty
   elective 62–3
   see also percutaneous transluminal coronary angioplasty
angiotensin-converting enzyme inhibitors see ACE inhibitors
angiotensin receptor blockers (ARBs)
   avoidance during pregnancy 191

angiotensin receptor blockers (ARBs) – *continued*
  in dilated cardiomyopathy 145
  indications and contraindications 8
  in STEMI 42
anterior myocardial infarction
  ECG 39
  peri-infarct arrhythmia 55
antiarrhythmics, QT prolongation 132
antibiotic prophylaxis 105
  in tetralogy of Fallot 173
antibiotics
  in bacterial endocarditis 103–4
  QT prolongation 132
anticoagulation
  after cardioversion 116
  in atrial fibrillation 116, 141
    RE-LY study 119
  in impaired systolic function 145
  and infective endocarditis 105
  during pregnancy 187
antidepressants, QT prolongation 132
antihypertensive treatment 11
  aliskiren 10
  whilst breastfeeding 193
  choice of agent 7–10
  in hypertensive urgency 71–2
  indications 3, 5
  parenteral 72
  during pregnancy 190–2
antiplatelet agents 24
  in NSTEMI 33, 35–6
  in secondary prevention 61
  in STEMI 38
antipsychotics, QT prolongation 132
antithrombotic therapy, in NSTEMI 33
aortic dissection
  classification 66, 67
  clinical presentation 65–6
  complications 66–7, 68
  CT appearance 67
  diagnosis 66, 69
  management 67–70, 69
    endovascular stents 69
    hypertension 73
aortic regurgitation
  associated murmurs 79
  asymptomatic 98–9
  clinical presentation 97
  investigation 97–8
  management 98–9
aortic stenosis
  clinical presentation 92
  investigation 93–4
  left ventricular hypertrophy 93
  management 94–5
  percutaneous valve implantation 96
  poor left ventricular function 96
aortic valve, bicuspid 175
aortic valve repair 99
aortic valve replacement (AVR) 99
  in aortic regurgitation 98
  in aortic stenosis 95
  conduction abnormalities 127
apixaban 119
ARBITER 6-HALTS trial 16
arrhythmias 21
  after surgery for tetralogy of Fallot 173
  atrial fibrillation
    classification 114
    clinical presentation 113
    management 114–17
  in atrial septal defects 166
  bradyarrhythmia
    clinical presentation 126
    management 127–9
  broad complex tachycardia
    clinical presentation 120
    ECG 120–1
    management 121–5
  in dilated cardiomyopathy 145
  investigation of palpitations 107–8
  narrow complex tachycardia
    causes 108–10
    clinical presentation 107, 108
    management 110–12
  peri-infarct 54, 58
    conduction abnormalities 54–5
    implantable cardioverter defibrillators 58
    supraventricular tachycardias 57–8
    ventricular arrhythmias 56–7
  pregnancy risk 178
  sudden cardiac death
    clinical presentation 131
    congenital long QT syndromes 133
    investigation 133
    sudden death syndromes 134
arrhythmogenic right ventricular dysplasia 134
ASCOT (Anglo-Scandinavian Cardiac Outcomes Trial) 8
  Lipid Lowering Arm 1–2, 6
aspirin
  effect on pre-eclampsia risk 190
  high dose in pericarditis 155
  in NSTEMI 33
  in secondary prevention 61
  in stable angina 24
  in STEMI 38
atenolol
  during pregnancy 185
  see also beta-blockers
ATHENA trial 118
athletes, screening for cardiovascular disease 134

atorvastatin
  after MI 61
  in primary prevention (ASCOT-LLA) 1–2
  see also statins
atrial fibrillation
  causes 114
  classification 114
  clinical presentation 113
  in dilated cardiomyopathy 145
  ECG 113–14
  in hypertrophic cardiomyopathy 141
  investigation 114
  management
    anti-arrhythmic drugs 117
    anticoagulation 116, 119
    DC cardioversion 115–16
    dronedarone 118
    medical 114–15
    pharmacological cardioversion 116
    radiofrequency ablation 117, 119
  management algorithm 115
  in mitral regurgitation 87, 88, 89, 91
  in mitral stenosis 83, 85
  peri-infarct 57–8
  during pregnancy 185
  recurrent
    management algorithm 118
  in restrictive cardiomyopathy 150
atrial flutter
  ECG 110
  LADIP study 112
atrial myxoma
  associated murmurs 79
  clinical features 80
  clinical presentation 79
  echocardiography 80, 81
  investigation 80
  management 81
atrial septal defect (ASD)
  adult presentation 166–7
  classification 166
  clinical presentation 165, 166–7
  clinical signs 167
  closure device, X-ray appearance 169
  indications for closure 167–8
  investigation 165–6, 167
  long-term complications 168
  management algorithm 168
  pregnancy risk 178
  in tetralogy of Fallot 171
atrioventricular nodal re-entry tachycardia
    (AVNRT) 108
  management 110
atropine
  in bradyarrhythmias 127, 130
  in peri-infarct arrhythmias 54

autoantibodies, in dilated cardiomyopathy 146
autonomic neuropathy, in AL amyloidosis 150
AV re-entry tachycardia (AVRT) 108
  management 110

barrier methods of contraception 179
Bazett formula 132
BEAUTIFUL trial 26
benign tumours 81
benzylpenicillin, in bacterial endocarditis 103
beta-blockers
  in atrial fibrillation 58, 115
  in dilated cardiomyopathy 145
  in hypertension 72, 73
    indications and contraindications 8–9
  in hypertrophic cardiomyopathy 139
  in NSTEMI 33
  perioperative 196–7
  during pregnancy 185
  in secondary prevention 61–2
  in stable angina 25
  in STEMI 42
  in termination of supraventricular tachycardias
    110
  use during pregnancy 191, 192
  in vasovagal syncope 76
  in ventricular tachycardias 56, 122, 123
bicuspid aortic valve 99, 175
bioprosthetic heart valves 188
Blalock–Taussig shunt 172
bleeding complications, PCI 45, 47
blood cultures, diagnosis of infective endocarditis
    102–3
blood pressure
  classification 7
  control in aortic dissection 68
  exercise response 21
  indications for antihypertensive treatment
    3, 5
  target levels 9, 10
    after MI 61
    during pregnancy 192, 193
  see also hypertension
bradyarrhythmia
  clinical presentation 126
  management 127–9
  after MI 46
  see also complete heart block
breastfeeding
  antihypertensive treatment 193
  warfarin 187
broad complex tachycardia
  clinical presentation 120
  ECG 120–1
  investigation 121–2
  management 121

broad complex tachycardia – *continued*
  management – *continued*
    implantable cardioverter defibrillators 122–3
    medical 122
    radiofrequency ablation 124, 125
Brugada syndrome 134

C-reactive protein (CRP), highly-sensitive 16
calcium channel blockers
  ALLHAT 7–8
  in atrial fibrillation 115
  indications and contraindications 8
  in NSTEMI 35
  in stable angina 26
  in supraventricular tachycardias 110, 111
Canadian Cardiovascular Society
  classification of angina symptom severity 18, 19
CAPRIE (Clopidogrel versus Aspirin in Patients at Risk of Ischaemic Events) trial 61
cardiac arrest, UK Resuscitation Council Guidelines 57
cardiac catheterization, differentiation between restriction and constriction 149
cardiac magnetic resonance imaging *see* magnetic resonance imaging
cardiac output, changes during pregnancy 184
cardiac resynchronization therapy, in dilated cardiomyopathy 146
cardiac tamponade
  clinical features 157, 160
  echocardiography 158–9
  management 159
cardiac tumours 80–1
  differentiation from thrombi 81
  see also atrial myxoma
cardiogenic shock 48
  causes 49
  management
    general 49, 53
    inotropic support 51
    intra-aortic balloon pumps 51–2
    nitric oxide synthase inhibitors 53
    oxygenation 49
    percutaneous left ventricular assist devices 53
    pulmonary artery catheterization 50–1
    renal support 52
    revascularization 52
  management algorithm 50
cardiomyopathy
  peripartum 183–4
  see also dilated cardiomyopathy; hypertrophic cardiomyopathy (HCM); restrictive cardiomyopathy

cardioversion
  atrial fibrillation 57–8, 115–16
  ventricular tachycardia 56
carpal tunnel syndrome, in AL amyloidosis 150
Carpentier–Edwards porcine prosthesis 188
CAST (Cardiac Arrhythmia Suppression Trials) 55
catecholamine crisis, treatment of hypertension 73
catecholaminergic polymorphic ventricular tachycardia 134
chemotherapy, in AL amyloidosis 150
chest pain, differential diagnosis 65–6
chest X-ray
  appearance of pacemakers and ICDs 124
  in coarctation of aorta 174
chlorthalidone, ALLHAT 7–8
chronic obstructive pulmonary disease, and beta-blockers 62
clopidogrel
  in NSTEMI 33, 35
  in secondary prevention 61
  in stable angina 24
  in STEMI 38
coarctation of aorta
  associated abnormalities 175
  clinical presentation 174, 175
  complications of surgical repair 176
  investigation 174–5
  long-term complications 175
  percutaneous balloon angioplasty 176
  surgical treatment 176
colchicine, in pericarditis 155
combined oral contraceptives, use by women with heart disease 179
COMMIT (Clopidogrel and Metoprolol in Myocardial Infarction Trial) 38, 42
complete heart block
  causes 127
  ECG 126–7
  initial assessment 127
  after MI 55
  permanent pacing 128–30
  temporary pacing 127–8
computed tomography
  in coarctation of aorta 175
  multislice in mitral stenosis 86
conduction abnormalities
  causes 127
  in restrictive cardiomyopathy 150
  see also complete heart block; heart block
congenital heart disease
  contraceptive methods 178
  maternal risk of pregnancy 177–8
  see also atrial septal defect (ASD); coarctation of aorta; tetralogy of Fallot; ventricular septal defect (VSD)
congenital long QT syndromes 133

constrictive pericarditis
  differentiation from restrictive cardiomyopathy 148–9, 151
  ventricular interdependence 151
contraception, women with heart disease 178–80
COPE (Colchicine for Acute Pericarditis) study 155
CORE (Colchicine for Recurrent Pericarditis) study 155
coronary angiography 22
  before aortic valve replacement 95, 98
  in atrial myxoma 81
  CT 23
  in aortic dissection 66
  in NSTEMI 35
  prior to surgery 197, 199
  right coronary artery occlusion and angioplasty 38
coronary artery bypass grafting (CABG) 62–3
  in stable angina 24, 27, 28, 29
  see also revascularization
coronary artery stenosis, risk of acute coronary syndrome 22–3
coronary care units 38
COURAGE (Clinical Outcomes Utilizing Revascularization and Aggressive Drug Evaluation) trial 28–9
CURE (Clopidogrel in Unstable Angina to Prevent Recurrent Events) trial 33, 61
cyanosis, in tetralogy of Fallot 171
cyanotic heart disease
  contraception 179
  pregnancy risk 178

dabigatran, in atrial fibrillation 119
DANAMI (Danish Trial in Acute Myocardial Infarction)-2 43
De Bakey classification, aortic dissection 66, 67
delta waves 108–9
Depo Provera 180
diabetes mellitus
  ACCORD trial 10
  ADVANCE study 10
  glycaemic control after MI 60–1
  lipid lowering therapy 6, 13–14
  management after STEMI 42–3
  risk from antihypertensive therapy 9
diamorphine
  in NSTEMI 35
  in STEMI 38
diastolic murmurs 79
  investigation 80
diet 59
DIGAMI (Diabetes Mellitus Insulin-Glucose Infusion in Acute Myocardial Infarction) study 60

DiGeorge syndrome, heart defects 166
digoxin
  in atrial fibrillation 115
  in restrictive cardiomyopathy 150
  in supraventricular tachycardias 111
dilated cardiomyopathy
  autoantibodies 146
  biventricular pacing 146
  causes 145
  clinical presentation 142
  treatment 144–5
  ventricular arrhythmias 145
  ventricular assist devices 146
diltiazem
  in atrial fibrillation 115
  in NSTEMI 35
  during pregnancy 185
  in stable angina 26
DINAMIT (Defibrillator in Acute Myocardial Infarction Trial) 58
dipyridamole, in stress testing 20
direct renin inhibitors 10
disopyramide
  in atrial fibrillation 117
  in hypertrophic cardiomyopathy 140
  in vasovagal syncope 76, 77
diuretics
  in dilated cardiomyopathy 144–5
  during pregnancy 185, 192
  in restrictive cardiomyopathy 150
dobutamine
  in cardiogenic shock 51
  stress testing 20
    pre-operative 196
dopamine, in cardiogenic shock 51
Doppler echocardiography
  in aortic stenosis 93, 94
  in coarctation of aorta 175
Down syndrome, heart defects 166
doxazosin, ALLHAT 7–8
dronedarone 118
drug-eluting stents 28
  non-cardiac surgery 197–8
dual chamber pacing 128, 129
  in hypertrophic cardiomyopathy 140
Duke criteria, infective endocarditis 102
dyslipidaemia
  rimonabant 15
  treatment guidelines 13–16

ECG
  prior to athletic training 134
  atrial fibrillation 113–14
  atrial flutter 110
  in atrial septal defects 166, 167
  broad complex tachycardia 120–1

ECG – *continued*
  complete heart block 126–7
  in hypertension 71
  idioventricular rhythm 55
  in inferior myocardial infarction 39
  left ventricular hypertrophy and strain 93
  localization of MI 39
  narrow complex tachycardia 108
  in NSTEMI 30, 32
  in pericardial effusion 157–8
  in pericarditis 153, 154
  pre-excitation 109
  QT prolongation 131
  right ventricular outflow tract VT 125
  sinus pause 76
  in stable angina 18–19
  in STEMI 37
  stress testing 20–1
  in syncope 75
  torsades de pointes 131
  in ventricular septal defect 162
  ventricular tachycardia 56
echocardiography
  in aortic dissection 66
  in aortic regurgitation 97
  in aortic stenosis 93–4
  atrial appendage thrombus 114
  in atrial myxoma 80
  in atrial septal defects 166, 167
  in coarctation of aorta 175
  diastolic murmurs, investigation of 80
  in dilated cardiomyopathy 144
  in hypertrophic cardiomyopathy 138
  in infective endocarditis 101–2, 103
  in mitral regurgitation 88, 89, 91
  in mitral stenosis 84–5
  in pericardial effusion 154–5, 158–9
  in restrictive cardiomyopathy 147–8
  in stable angina 19
  stress testing 21
  after tetralogy of Fallot repair 171
  in ventricular septal defect 162
  in ventricular tachycardias 122
EGSYS (Evaluation of Guidelines in Syncope Study) 75
Eisenmenger's syndrome 163
ejection systolic murmurs 165, 167, 174
electrocardiography *see* ECG
elderly people, antihypertensive treatment 10
enalapril, in aortic regurgitation 98
endocardial cushion VSDs 162
endomyocardial biopsy 143, 146
  in amyloidosis 149
endovascular stents, in aortic dissection 68, 69
enoxaparin, in NSTEMI 33
enterococcal endocarditis 103

EPHESUS (Eplerenone Post-Acute Myocardial Infarction Heart Failure Efficacy and Survival Study) 42, 62
epidural anaesthesia, in mitral stenosis 185
eplerenone
  in secondary prevention 62
  in STEMI 42
eptifibatide, in NSTEMI 33
essential hypertension 174
EUROPA (EUropean trial on Reduction Of cardiac events with Perindopril in stable coronary Artery disease) 27, 62
exercise after MI 59–60
exercise testing 20
  in aortic regurgitation 97–8
  in aortic stenosis 94
  in heart failure 143–4
  in hypertrophic cardiomyopathy 140
  in mitral regurgitation 89
  pre-operative 196, 199
  see also stress testing
external pacing 127–8
ezetimibe 14

Fallot's tetralogy *see* tetralogy of Fallot
familial dilated cardiomyopathy with atrioventricular block 134
fenofibrate 14
  combination with statins 15
fibrates 14–15
  indications and contraindications 15
fibroelastomas 81
FINESSE (Facilitated Intervention with Enhanced Reperfusion Speed to Stop Events) study 43
fish oils 15
flecainide
  in atrial fibrillation 117
  in peri-infarct arrhythmias 55
  pharmacological cardioversion 116
  in supraventricular tachycardias 111
flucloxacillin, in bacterial endocarditis 103
fludrocortisone, in vasovagal syncope 76–7
fluid overload 147
fluoxetine, in vasovagal syncope 76
folic acid supplementation after MI 64
Fontan circulation
  contraception 180
  pregnancy risk 178
  risks of laparoscopy 180
FRISC (Fragmin during Instability in Coronary Artery Disease) study 32, 62
furosemide in hypertensive emergencies 72

gentamicin, in bacterial endocarditis 103
gestational hypertension 189–90
  management 191

giant cell myocarditis 143
GISSI (Gruppo Italiano per lo Studio della Sopravvivenza nell'Infarto Miocardico) 61
glitazones (thiazolidinediones) 61
global CVD risk 2, 6
glycaemic control after MI 42–3, 60–1
glyceryl trinitrate (GTN)
   in hypertensive emergencies 72
   in NSTEMI 35
GRACE (Global Registry of Acute Coronary Events) score 31
graft patency, long-term, CABG 28
Graham–Steell murmur 79
'granular sparkling' pattern, cardiac amyloidosis 148

HbA1c, target levels after MI 60–1
heart block
   after MI 46
   after percutaneous VSD closure 164
   see also complete heart block
heart failure
   initial management 142
   investigation 142–4
   during pregnancy
      causes 183–4
      investigation 184
      management 185
heart rate correction, QT interval 132
heparin
   in NSTEMI 33
   during pregnancy 187
   in STEMI 39–40
hepatomegaly
   in AL amyloidosis 150
high-density lipoprotein (HDL) cholesterol
   as therapeutic target 14
highly-sensitive C-reactive protein
   JUPITER trial 16
homografts 188
HOPE (Heart Outcomes Prevention Evaluation) study 27
hydralazine
   in hypertensive emergencies 72
   use during pregnancy 192
hypertension 11
   ACCORD trial 10
   ADVANCE study 10
   choice of antihypertensive agent 8–10
   clinical assessment 70
   combination therapy 10
   in elderly people 10
   essential 174
   grading 7
   investigations 70–1
   management after MI 61

   during pregnancy 189–90
      blood pressure targets 192, 193
      management 190–2
      postpartum management 192–3
      risks 190
   secondary causes 174
   threshold for intervention 3, 5
   treatment algorithm 9
hypertensive emergencies 71
   survival 73
   treatment 72–3
hypertensive retinopathy
   Keith–Wagner classification 71
hypertensive urgency 71
   treatment 71–2
hypertrophic cardiomyopathy (HCM)
   atrial fibrillation 141
   clinical presentation 137
   diagnosis 138
   implantable cardioverter defibrillators 140–1
   inheritance 138
   management 138–9
      medical 139–40
      surgical 140
   myocardial fibrosis 141
   pregnancy risk 178
   risk of sudden death 140
   risk stratification 140–1
   symptoms 138–9
hypokalemia 58
   QT prolongation 132
hypomagnesaemia 58
   QT prolongation 132
hypotension
   after MI
      causes 45
      investigation 45–6
      management 46
   in AL amyloidosis 150
   in cardiogenic shock 48
HYVET (Hypertension in the Very Elderly Trial) 10

idioventricular rhythm 55–6
Implanon 180
implantable cardioverter defibrillators 56, 58, 121, 122–3
   chest X-ray appearance 124
   in dilated cardiomyopathy 145, 146
   in hypertrophic cardiomyopathy 140–1
   NICE guidelines 63
implantable loop recorders, in investigation of syncope 75, 77–8
infective endocarditis
   antibiotic prophylaxis 105
   clinical presentation 100

infective endocarditis – *continued*
  culture-negative 103
  diagnosis 101–3
  indications for surgery 104
  risk from intrauterine devices 180
  risk in tetralogy of Fallot 173
  treatment 103–5
inferior myocardial infarction
  arrhythmias 54–5
  ECG 39
inotropic support in cardiogenic shock 51
INSTEAD (INvestigation of StEnt Grafts in Patients with type B Aortic Dissection) study 69
insulin resistance, changes during pregnancy 184
insulin therapy after STEMI 42–3
International Diabetes Federation, definition of metabolic syndrome 12
intra-aortic balloon pumps, in cardiogenic shock 51–2
intracranial aneurysms, association with coarctation of aorta 175
intravenous fluids, increasing left ventricular filling pressure 46
ion channel abnormalities 133
IONA (Impact of Nicorandil in Angina) study 26
ischaemic heart disease
  mitral regurgitation 91
  see also angina; myocardial infarction; non-ST elevation myocardial infarction; ST elevation myocardial infarction
ISIS-2 (Second International Study of Infarct Survival) 38
ISSUE (International Study on Syncope of Uncertain Etiology) 2 77–8
ivabradine, in stable angina 26

JBS (Joint British Societies), guidelines for primary prevention 2
jugular venous pressure 160
  in cardiac tamponade 160
JUPITER (Justification for the Use of statins in Prevention: an Intervention Trial Evaluating Rosuvastatin) 16

Keith–Wagner classification, hypertensive retinopathy 71
Killip classification, acute myocardial infarction 42

labetolol
  in hypertensive emergencies 72, 73
  use during pregnancy 192
LADIP (Loire–Ardèche–Drôme–Isère–Puy-de-Dôme) study 112

laparoscopy, risks in women with congenital heart disease 180
left bundle branch block 19
left ventricular filling pressure, raising with IV fluids 46
left ventricular hypertrophy 19
  in aortic stenosis 93
  ECG 93
  in hypertrophic cardiomyopathy 138
left ventricular outflow tract obstruction 138
  surgical intervention 140
lifestyle modification 13
  after MI 59–60
lignocaine, in peri-infarct arrhythmias 56
lipid levels, monitoring 1–2
lipid lowering therapy
  after MI 61
  guidelines 13–16
  in primary prevention 1–2, 6, 13
  in stable angina 27
lipomas 81
lisinopril, ALLHAT 7–8
loss of consciousness, assessment 77
low molecular weight heparins
  in NSTEMI 33
  during pregnancy 187, 188
low-density lipoprotein cholesterol, target levels 2, 13, 27, 61
lymphomas 81

macroglossia, in AL amyloidosis 150
MADIT (Multicenter Automatic Defibrillator Implantation Trial) 123
magnetic resonance imaging (MRI) 143, 144
  in amyloidosis 149
  in aortic regurgitation 97
  in atrial myxoma 81
  in atrial septal defects 167
  in coarctation of aorta 175
  stress testing 22, 23
  after tetralogy of Fallot repair 171–2
  in ventricular septal defect 162
  in ventricular tachycardias 122
malignant pericardial effusions 159
malignant tumours 81
Marfan syndrome, pregnancy risk 178
mechanical heart valves
  contraception 179
  pregnancy
    anticoagulation 187
    risk 178
MERLIN (Metabolic Efficiency with Ranolazine for Less Ischaemia in Non-ST elevation myocardial infarction) trial 26
metabolic syndrome 12–13

lipid lowering therapy 13–14
metastatic tumours 81
metformin, interaction with intravenous contrast 43
methyldopa, use during pregnancy 192
metoprolol
  in NSTEMI 33
  perioperative use 197
  during pregnancy 185
  in STEMI 42
midodrine, in vasovagal syncope 76
migraine, association with patent foramen ovale 169–70
milrinone, in cardiogenic shock 51
Mirena intrauterine device 180
MIST (Migraine Intervention with STARFlex Technology) trial 169–70
mitral regurgitation
  atrial fibrillation 91
  clinical assessment 87–8
  clinical presentation 87
  investigation 88–9, 91
  ischaemic 91
  management 89–91
  severity 88
mitral stenosis 85
  associated murmurs 79
  atrial fibrillation 85
  causes 84
  clinical presentation 83
  investigation 84–5
  management algorithm 86
  multislice computed tomography 86
  percutaneous balloon valvotomy 85
  during pregnancy
    clinical presentation 183
    effect of physiological changes 184
    management 185
    management of delivery 185–6
    risks 184–5
  rheumatic
    natural history 84
  Wilkins score 85
mitral valve
  abnormalities in coarctation of aorta 175
  systolic anterior motion (SAM) 138
mitral valve surgery
  indications 89
  during pregnancy 185
  types of procedure 89–90
Morrow procedure 140
murmurs
  diastolic 79–80
  ejection systolic 165, 167, 174
  pansystolic 161
muscular VSDs 162, 163

myocardial fibrosis, in hypertrophic cardiomyopathy 141
myocardial infarction
  implantable cardioverter defibrillators 63
  perioperative
    beta-blocker prophylaxis 196–7
    risk assessment 195–6, 198–9
  secondary prevention
    ACE (angiotensin-converting enzyme) inhibitors) 62
    aldosterone receptor antagonists 62
    antiplatelet agents 61
    beta-blockers 61–2
    blood pressure control 61
    elective angioplasty 62–3
    glycaemic control 60–1
    lifestyle modification 59–60
    lipid lowering therapy 61
    vitamin and folic acid supplements 64
  see also non-ST elevation myocardial infarction; ST elevation myocardial infarction
myocardial ischaemia
  assessment 20–2
  induction 20
myopericarditis 155
myositis, risk in statin therapy 15
myxoma see atrial myxoma

narrow complex tachycardia
  causes 108–10
  ECG 108
  management 110–11
    LADIP study 112
nephrotic syndrome in AL amyloidosis 150
NICE (National Institute for Health and Clinical Excellence)
  guidelines for automatic implantable cardioverter defibrillators 63
  guidelines for lipid lowering therapy 13
nicorandil
  in NSTEMI 35
  in stable angina 26
nicotinic acid (niacin) 14–15
  ARBITER 6-HALTS trial 16
  combination with statins 15
  indications and contraindications 15
nifedipine
  in aortic regurgitation 98
  in stable angina 26
  sublingual 72–3
  use during pregnancy 192
nitrates
  intravenous 73
  in NSTEMI 33, 35
  in stable angina 26

nitric oxide synthase inhibitors, in cardiogenic shock 53
non-ST elevation myocardial infarction (NSTEMI) 30–1
  clinical presentation 29
  diagnostic algorithm 31
  management 33–5
    antiplatelet agents 35–6
  risk stratification 31–3
  see also myocardial infarction
non-steroidal anti-inflammatory drugs (NSAIDs)
  in pericarditis 155

obesity 59
omega-3 fatty acids, benefits after MI 61
opiates
  in NSTEMI 35
  in STEMI 38
oral contraception, use by women with heart disease 179
orthostatic hypotension
  causes 75
  treatment 76
ostium primum ASD 166
outlet septum type VSDs 162
oxygen therapy in cardiogenic shock 49

PACE (Promoting Healthy Ageing with Cognitive Exercise) study 129
pacemaker syndrome 129
pacemakers
  chest X-ray appearance 124
  in dilated cardiomyopathy 146
  in hypertrophic cardiomyopathy 140
  nomenclature 128
  in peri-infarct arrhythmias 54, 55
  permanent 128–30
  temporary 127–8
  in vasovagal syncope 77
palpitations
  investigation 107–8
  see also arrhythmias
pansystolic murmur
  causes 161
  investigation 161–2
papillary fibroelastomas 81
paradoxical emboli
  in atrial septal defects 166–7
  in patent foramen ovale 169
patent foramen ovale (PFO)
  association with stroke 169
  trial of closure 169–70
pentalogy of Fallot 171
percutaneous alcohol septal ablation 140
percutaneous aortic valve surgery 95, 96

percutaneous balloon angioplasty, in coarctation of aorta 176
percutaneous balloon mitral valvuloplasty 85, 185, 186
percutaneous left ventricular assist devices 53
percutaneous transluminal coronary angioplasty (PTCA)
  bleeding complications 45, 47
  prior to surgery 197–8
  in stable angina 24, 27–8, 29
  in STEMI 39, 43
  see also revascularization
percutaneous VSD closure 164
pericardial effusions
  clinical presentation 157
  drainage 159
  ECG changes 157–8
  echocardiography 158–9
  investigation 154–5
  management 159–60
  recurrence 159
pericardial rub 153–4
pericarditis
  causes 154
  clinical presentation 153–4
  constrictive
    differentiation from restrictive cardiomyopathy 148–9, 151
    ventricular interdependence 151
  ECG 153, 154
  high-risk features 155, 156
  investigation 154–5
  treatment 155–6
perimembranous VSDs 162, 163
perindopril
  EUROPA trial 27, 62
  see also ACE (angiotensin-converting enzyme) inhibitors
perindopril–indapamide combination
  ADVANCE study 10
perioperative beta-blockers 196–7
perioperative risk stratification 195–6, 198–9
peripartum cardiomyopathy 183–4
peripheral vascular disease, and beta-blockers 62
permanent pacing 128–30
phaeochromocytoma, hypertensive emergency 73
pharmacological cardioversion, atrial fibrillation 116
pharmacological stress tests
  pre-operative 196
  see also stress testing
phentolamine, in hypertensive emergencies 72
phosphodiesterase inhibitors, in cardiogenic shock 51
'pill in the pocket' medication, atrial fibrillation 117

plasma cell dyscrasias, AL amyloidosis 150
plasma volume, changes during pregnancy 184
POISE (Perioperative Ischaemia Evaluation) trial 197
POST (Prevention of Syncope Trial) 76
potassium channel agonists
  in NSTEMI 35
  in stable angina 26
Potts shunt 172
PR segment depression, in pericarditis 153, 154
prasugrel 35–6
pravastatin, in primary prevention 13
pre-eclampsia 190
  management 191, 192
pre-excitation 108, 109
pregnancy
  hypertension 189–90
    blood pressure targets 192, 193
    management 190–2
    postpartum management 192–3
    risks 190
  mechanical heart valves
    anticoagulation 187
  mitral stenosis
    clinical presentation 183
    effect of physiological changes 184
    management 185
    management of delivery 185–6
    risks 184–5
  pre-conception counselling 187
  risks in congenital heart disease 177–8
pre-hospital thrombolysis 41
primary percutaneous coronary intervention (PPCI) 39, 43
primary prevention 8–10
  antihypertensive treatment 7–10
  blood pressure 3, 5
  CVD risk charts 3–4
  global CVD risk 2, 6
  JBS guidelines 2
  lipid lowering therapy 1–2, 6, 13
primum ASD 166
  closure 168
progestogen-only contraception, use by women with heart disease 179–80
propafenone
  in atrial fibrillation 117
  pharmacological cardioversion 116
  in supraventricular tachycardias 111
prosthetic valves
  bioprosthetic 188
  pregnancy
    anticoagulation 187
  staphylococcal infection 103
pulmonary atresia 171
pulmonary hypertension, pregnancy risk 178

pulmonary regurgitation
  associated murmurs 79
  after tetralogy of Fallot repair 172–3
pulmonary stenosis, percutaneous techniques 173
pulmonary wedge pressure 46
  in cardiogenic shock 50–1
pulsus paradoxus 157, 160
purpura, periorbital in AL amyloidosis 150

Q waves, in stable angina 18–19
QT interval 132
QT prolongation 131–2, 134
  causes 132–3
  congenital long QT syndromes 133

radial artery access, coronary interventions 45, 47
radiofrequency ablation 110
  in atrial fibrillation 117, 119
  LADIP study 112
  in ventricular tachycardias 124
radionuclide scintigraphy 22
radionuclide ventriculography in aortic regurgitation 97
RALES (Randomized Aldosterone Evaluation Study) 62
ramipril
  HOPE study 27
  in secondary prevention 62
  in STEMI 42
  see also ACE (angiotensin-converting enzyme) inhibitors
ranolazine, in stable angina 26
REACT (Rescue Angioplasty Versus Conservative Treatment or Repeat Thrombolysis) trial 41
re-entry tachycardias 108
RE-LY study 119
renal impairment in hypertensive emergencies 73
renal support in cardiogenic shock 52
reperfusion therapy
  failure 41
  idioventricular rhythm 55–6
  indications 38–9
  see also primary percutaneous coronary intervention (PPCI); thrombolysis
rescue angioplasty 41
restenosis after PCA 28
restrictive cardiomyopathy
  causes 148
  clinical presentation 147
  differentiation from constrictive pericarditis 148–9, 151
  echocardiography 147–8
  treatment 150

resuscitation, UK Resuscitation Council
   Guidelines 57
reteplase, in facilitation of PCI 43
retinopathy, hypertensive, Keith–Wagner
   classification 71
revascularization
   in cardiogenic shock 52
   in NSTEMI 35
   see also coronary artery bypass grafting
      (CABG); percutaneous transluminal
      coronary angioplasty
Revised Cardiac Risk Index (RCRI) 196
rhabdomyolysis risk, statin therapy 15
rhabdomyomas 81
rheumatic heart disease 84, 86, 94
rifampicin in bacterial endocarditis 103
right bundle branch block, in atrial septal defects
   167
right ventricular infarcts, hypotension 45
right ventricular outflow tract VT 124
   ECG 125
rimonabant 15
risk stratification 6
   blood pressure 3, 5
   CVD risk charts 3–4
   lipid levels 1–2
   metabolic syndrome 12–13
   stress echocardiography 21
rivaroxaban 119
rosiglitazone 61
Ross procedure 188
rosuvastatin
   JUPITER trial 16
   see also statins

sarcoma 81
SAVE PACE (Search AV Extension and Managed
   Ventricular Pacing for Promoting
   Atrioventricular Conduction) study 130
Scandinavian Simvastatin Survival Study (4S) 61
SCD-HEFT (Sudden Cardiac Death in Heart
   Failure Trial) 123
secondary hypertension 174
secondary prevention
   ACE (angiotensin-converting enzyme)
      inhibitors) 62
   aldosterone receptor antagonists 62
   antiplatelet agents 61
   beta-blockers 61–2
   blood pressure control 61
   elective angioplasty 62–3
   glycaemic control 60–1
   lifestyle modification 59–60
   lipid lowering therapy 61
   vitamin and folic acid supplements 64
secundum ASD 166

closure 168, 169
selective serotonin reuptake inhibitors (SSRIs), in
   vasovagal syncope 76
SHOCK (SHould we emergently revascularize
   Occluded Coronaries for shocK) trial 49, 52
simvastatin
   4S (Scandinavian Simvastatin Survival Study)
      61
   in primary prevention 13, 16
   see also statins
single chamber pacing 128–9
sinus pause 76
sinus venosus defects 166
   closure 168
smoking cessation 59
sodium nitroprusside 72–3
   in aortic dissection 68
   use during pregnancy 192
sotalol
   in atrial fibrillation 117
   in supraventricular tachycardias 111
South Asian origin, coronary disease risk 13
SPECT (single photon emission computed
   tomography) 22
spironolactone
   avoidance during pregnancy 191
   in dilated cardiomyopathy 145
   in secondary prevention 62
ST depression
   in stable angina 18–19
   in stress testing 20
ST elevation
   as indicator of extent of myocardial risk 38–9
   in pericarditis 153, 154
ST elevation myocardial infarction (STEMI)
   ACE (angiotensin-converting enzyme)
      inhibitors 42
   aldosterone receptor antagonists 42
   angiotensin receptor blockers 42
   arrhythmias 54–5, 58
      conduction abnormalities 54–5
      implantable cardioverter defibrillators 58
      supraventricular tachycardias 57–8
      ventricular 55–6
   beta-blockers 42
   cardiogenic shock 48
      management 49–53
   clinical presentation 36–7
   diabetes management 42–3
   diagnostic algorithm 31
   ECG 37
   failed reperfusion 41
   hypotension 44–5
      causes 45
      investigation 45–6
      management 46

initial management 37–8, 43–4
Killip classification 42
localization 39
management algorithm 40
mortality risk 59
reperfusion therapy
   indications 38–9
   PPCI 39, 43
   thrombolysis 39–41
   see also myocardial infarction
Stanford classification, aortic dissection 66, 67
staphylococcal endocarditis 103
statins
   in aortic stenosis 94–5
   combination with other lipid lowering agents 15
   indications and contraindications 15
   after MI 61
   pleiotropic effects 61
   in primary prevention 1–2, 13, 16
   in secondary prevention 27
stent thrombosis, arrhythmias 56
stenting
   in coarctation of aorta 176
   prior to surgery 197–8
   in stable angina 28
sterilization, female 180
steroids, in pericarditis 155–6
streptococcal endocarditis 103
streptokinase, combination with aspirin in STEMI 38
stress testing
   in aortic regurgitation 97–8
   in aortic stenosis 94
   contraindications 22
   in mitral regurgitation 89
   pre-operative 196, 199
   in stable angina 19, 20–1
stroke
   in atrial septal defects 166–7
   in patent foramen ovale 169
   treatment of hypertension 73
subclavian steal syndrome 75
sudden cardiac death
   athletes 134
   clinical presentation 131
   congenital long QT syndromes 133
   in dilated cardiomyopathy 145
   in hypertrophic cardiomyopathy 140
   investigation 133
   in repaired tetralogy of Fallot 173
sudden death syndromes 134
supraventricular tachycardias
   causes 108–10
   management 110–11
      LADIP study 112

surgical myomectomy 140
Svensson classification, aortic dissection 66, 67
syncope
   assessment 77
   causes 74, 75
   implantable loop recorders 77–8
   investigation 75
   sinus pause 76
   tilt testing 78
   treatment 76–7
SYNPACE (SYNcope and PACing) study 77
systolic anterior motion (SAM), mitral valve 138
systolic area index 151

tachycardia, ventricular, peri-infarct 56
technetium radionuclide scintigraphy 22
temporary pacing 127–8
tenecteplase 39
tetralogy of Fallot
   antibiotic prophylaxis 173
   complications 171–2
   features 171
   late complications
      clinical presentation 170–1
   late complications of surgery 172–3
      investigation 171
   pregnancy risk 178
   surgical procedures 172
thallium radionuclide scintigraphy 22
thiazide diuretics
   ALLHAT 7–8
   indications and contraindications 8
   use during pregnancy 192
thiazolidinediones (glitazones) 61
thromboembolism
   risk in atrial fibrillation 116–17
   risk after cardioversion 116
thrombolysis 39–41
   contraindications 41
   failure 41
   followed by angiography and PCI 43
tilarginine, in cardiogenic shock 53
tilt testing, in vasovagal syncope 77, 78
time-dependency, benefits of thrombolysis 40–1
TIMI (Thrombolysis in Myocardial Infarction)
   risk score 31–2
tirofiban, in NSTEMI 33
tissue plasminogen activator therapy 39
torsades de pointes 131–2
total cholesterol, target levels 2, 13, 27, 61
transfer for PPCI 39, 43
transient ischaemic attacks 74
transoesophageal echocardiography
   before cardioversion 116
   in infective endocarditis 101, 103
   in mitral regurgitation 88

transoesophageal echocardiography – *continued*
　　in ventricular tachycardias 122
　　see also echocardiography
transvenous temporary pacing 128
tricuspid regurgitation
　　after surgery for tetralogy of Fallot 172–3
　　associated murmurs 79
triglyceride lowering therapy 14–15
TRITON (TRial to assess Improvement in Therapeutic outcomes by optimising platelet iNhibition with prasugrel) TIMI-38 35–6
troponins 31, 36
　　in pericarditis 154
　　in risk stratification 31–2
　　in ventricular tachycardias 121–2
tuberculous pericarditis 154
Turner's syndrome, coarctation of aorta 175
T-wave inversion, in pericarditis 154

UKPDS (United Kingdom Prospective Diabetes Study) 60
unstable angina
　　diagnostic algorithm 31
　　distinction from NSTEMI 31
'upstream treatment', NSTEMI 33
uraemic pericarditis 155

vagal manoeuvres, in termination of supraventricular tachycardias 110
vaginal delivery 185
　　in mitral stenosis 185–6
valsartan
in STEMI 42
see also angiotensin receptor blockers
valve disease
　　during pregnancy
　　　　clinical presentation 183
　　　　effect of physiological changes 184
　　　　management 185
　　　　risks 184–5
　　see also mitral regurgitation; mitral stenosis; pulmonary regurgitation; pulmonary stenosis; tricuspid regurgitation
valve replacement surgery
　　postoperative pyrexia 100–1
　　see also aortic valve replacement (AVR)
vancomycin, in bacterial endocarditis 103
vascular access
　　temporary pacing 128
vasoconstrictors, in vasovagal syncope 76
vasodilators
　　in aortic dissection 68
　　in aortic regurgitation 98
　　in mitral regurgitation 89
vasovagal syncope 74, 78
　　treatment 76–7
ventilation, in cardiogenic shock 49
ventricular arrhythmias
　　after MI 55–6
　　after STEMI 38
　　after surgery for tetralogy of Fallot 173
　　in dilated cardiomyopathy 145
　　in stress testing 21
　　see also ventricular tachycardias
ventricular assist devices, in dilated cardiomyopathy 146
ventricular interdependence 151
ventricular septal defect (VSD)
　　association with coarctation of aorta 175
　　classification 162, 163
　　clinical presentation 161, 162–3
　　indications for closure 162–3
　　investigation 161–2
　　management algorithm 164
　　percutaneous closure techniques 164
　　pregnancy risk 178
ventricular tachycardias (VTs)
　　investigation 121–2
　　management 121
　　　　implantable cardioverter defibrillators 122–3
　　　　medical 122
　　　　radiofrequency ablation 124, 125
　　see also ventricular arrhythmias
verapamil
　　in atrial fibrillation 115
　　in hypertrophic cardiomyopathy 139–40
　　in NSTEMI 35
　　during pregnancy 185
　　in stable angina 26
viral myocarditis 143
viral pericarditis, diagnosis 154
vitamin supplements, after MI 64
VPS (Vasovagal Pacemaker Study) II 77

wall motion, stress responses 21
warfarin, during pregnancy 187
warfarin embryopathy 187
Waterson shunt 172
weight control 59
weight reduction, rimonabant 15
Wilkins score, mitral stenosis 85
Wolff–Parkinson–White syndrome 109
WOSCOPS (West of Scotland Coronary Prevention Study) 1